RODICAN'S ULTIMATE GUIDE TO GETTING INTO PHYSICIAN ASSISTANT SCHOOL

Notice

Medicine is an ever-changing science. As new research and clinical experience broaden our knowledge, changes in treatment and drug therapy are required. The author and the publisher of this work have checked with sources believed to be reliable in their efforts to provide information that is complete and generally in accord with the standards accepted at the time of publication. However, in view of the possibility of human error or changes in medical sciences, neither the author nor the publisher nor any other party who has been involved in the preparation or publication of this work warrants that the information contained herein is in every respect accurate or complete, and they disclaim all responsibility for any errors or omissions or for the results obtained from use of the information contained in this work. Readers are encouraged to confirm the information contained herein with other sources. For example and in particular, readers are advised to check the product information sheet included in the package of each drug they plan to administer to be certain that the information contained in this work is accurate and that changes have not been made in the recommended dose or in the contraindications for administration. This recommendation is of particular importance in connection with new or infrequently used drugs.

RODICAN'S ULTIMATE GUIDE TO GETTING INTO PHYSICIAN ASSISTANT SCHOOL

FIFTH EDITION

Andrew J. Rodican, PA-C
CareMedica
North Haven, Connecticut

New York Chicago San Francisco Athens London Madrid Mexico City
New Delhi Milan Singapore Sydney Toronto

Rodican's Ultimate Guide to Getting into Physician Assistant School, Fifth Edition

1 2 3 4 5 6 7 8 9   LCR   27 26 25 24 23 22

ISBN 978-1-264-27888-6
MHID 1-264-27888-8

This book was set in Sabon LT Std by MPS Limited.
The editor was Sydney Keen.
The production supervisor was Catherine Saggese.
Production management was provided by Anamika Singh, MPS Limited.

This book is printed on acid-free paper.

Library of Congress Cataloging-in-Publication Data

Names: Rodican, Andrew J. author.
Title: Rodican's ultimate guide to getting into physician assistant school
   / Andrew J. Rodican.
Other titles: Ultimate guide to getting into physician assistant school
Description: Fifth edition. | New York : McGraw Hill, [2022] | Summary:
   "This book shows readers how to navigate the application process for
   physician assistant school"—Provided by publisher.
Identifiers: LCCN 2021049782 (print) | LCCN 2021049783 (ebook) | ISBN
   9781264278886 (paperback ; alk. paper) | ISBN 9781264278893 (ebook)
Subjects: MESH: Physician Assistants—education | School Admission Criteria
   | Vocational Guidance | Interviews as Topic | United States
Classification: LCC R697.P45 (print) | LCC R697.P45 (ebook) | NLM W 21.5
   | DDC 610.73/7069—dc23/eng/20211101
LC record available at https://lccn.loc.gov/2021049782
LC ebook record available at https://lccn.loc.gov/2021049783

I dedicate this book to the memory of my best friend:

Richard J. Vining, II
April 29, 1952–April 29, 2021
May you rest in peace, my friend. We will never forget you.

Contents

Foreword

I still vividly remember the first time I met Andy Rodican, back in 2005. He joined a well-known local cardiology practice and worked alongside very skilled specialists in cardiovascular disease prevention, weight loss, and well-being. What struck me the most about Andy was his uncommon and contagious passion. Every day he would fully embrace his mission of transforming lives, enthusiastically engaging with patients, and always trying to make his healing role meaningful.

Andy created the most successful independent weight-loss practice in New England, establishing novel clinical protocols and commercial strategies that are still vital today, almost 15 years later, to the whole Bariatric Medicine industry.

The same striking passion has characterized pretty much all of Andy's life. At age 17, he served his country as a US Navy Corpsman, graduated from the Yale University School of Medicine Physician Associate Program in 1994, and has helped thousands of PA school applicants achieve success since 1996.

This book represents only the latest chapter of Andy Rodican's quest to pave the way to success for future generations of medical professionals.

Today, Andy Rodican continues to make a big difference in the lives and careers of countless future physician assistants, not only by giving them great and up to date insights on how to master the PA school admission process in an ever more competitive landscape but also by continuing to mentor a large number of PA students during their clinical rotations in our CareMedica offices with the same passion and unwavering dedication.

Every time I ask Andy, "How are you doing?" She invariably answers with a big smile, "I've never had it so good."

Fausto Petruzziello, MD
Assistant Professor of Medicine
Yale School of Medicine
CEO/Medical Director
CareMedica and the MEDICA Companies

Introduction

In this book, I will show you how to navigate the application process for PA school. The PA profession continues to grow, and the competition for acceptance is fierce. If you're looking for a distinct advantage over the competition, this book is for you.

Since 1996, I've helped thousands of PA school applicants achieve success. I graduated from the Yale University School of Medicine Physician Associate Program in 1994, serving for 3 years on Yale's admissions committee. I wrote the first edition of this book in 1997, and the book continued to rate 4.5 stars on Amazon through 2021. I've coached PA school applicants for over 24 years now, and I am a pioneer in the field. I've helped thousands of applicants achieve success, and I can help you too. I am incredibly passionate about the PA profession and assisting others in getting accepted to PA school. I often feel that I get more from giving back to the applicants I coach than they get from me.

Getting accepted to PA school is a highly competitive process. Reading this book will give you an edge over the competition by providing a comprehensive review of the PA profession and the application process. You will learn to avoid the most common pitfalls that many *vanilla* applicants make during the application process. You will also learn how to obtain the best letters of recommendation and why you must get your CASPA application in as soon as the cycle opens.

Rodican's Ultimate Guide to Getting into Physician Assistant School, Fifth Edition, formerly *The Ultimate Guide to Getting into Physician Assistant School*, Fourth Edition, is *the* top-ranked book for PA school applicants on Amazon.com.

I promise you this book will make all of the difference between an acceptance email and rejection. Purchasing this book sooner rather than later will save you a lot of time in the long run. So don't wait; buy this book right now!

The tips and tricks you're about to read have proven results. In addition, each chapter provides new information and secrets that will help you maximize your success AND get a leg up on the competition. If you follow my advice in this book, you may have a long and fulfilling career as a physician assistant in the future. You will learn to become the *perfect applicant*.

CHAPTER 1

So You Want to be a Physician Assistant

First of all, congratulations! By investing in this book, you've just taken your first step toward achieving your goal of becoming a physician assistant (PA) school student. Whether you're a reapplicant to PA school or a first-time applicant, this book is going to help you get focused and provide you with all of the information you'll need to conquer the PA school application, essay, and interview process. Armed with this information, you will have a wealth of knowledge to help you become the perfect applicant.

No doubt, being a PA will challenge your intelligence, patience, compassion, and prejudices. But the profession will also reward you emotionally and financially. As you learn about the expanding roles of PAs in the health care system and the continued growth of the profession, you will realize that PAs are an integral part of the future of health care. You are about to embark on a journey that will allow you to enter one of the hottest professions in the United States and have a bright future ahead.

In this chapter, I'm going to define the role of the PA, provide information on the history of the PA profession, and discuss the following:

- The definition of a PA
- The evolution of the PA profession
- The training of PAs
- The future of the PA profession

- Salaries for PAs
- Six reasons to become a PA versus a physician
- The PA scope of practice
- The six things PA programs look for in a competitive applicant

I've personally had a gratifying career as a PA, and I wouldn't have changed one thing along the way after practicing over two decades. I hope you are excited to begin your journey, so let's get started.

WHAT IS A PA?

If you would like the "official" definition of a PA, visit the American Academy of Physician Assistants (AAPA) website at aapa.org. And, while you're on the AAPA website, I strongly recommend that you consider joining as an affiliate member. The AAPA website provides a wealth of information both for PAs and PA school applicants.

In general, PAs are licensed health care professionals who practice medicine under the supervision of a licensed physician. PAs are considered "dependent" practitioners because of their relationship with a supervising physician. PAs practice in all 50 states and also have prescription writing privileges in all 50 states.

PAs work very autonomously in their designated field of practice, although the level of autonomy will vary from practice to practice. Don't expect to follow your supervising physician around by the proverbial "coattails." A physician who knows how to utilize PAs most effectively will expect you to work autonomously within the scope of the practice, carry your patient load, and use your diagnostic and critical thinking skills. In many situations, PAs may not even work in the exact physical location as their supervising physician, but they must always remain in telephone contact. Typically, PAs meet with their supervising physician at least once per week.

Some of the duties and responsibilities of the PA include:

- Taking a medical history
- Performing a medical examination
- Ordering diagnostic testing (lab studies, X-rays, MRIs, etc.)
- Formulating a diagnosis and treatment plan

- Writing prescriptions
- Counseling patients
- Discussing preventative medicine
- Performing yearly physical examinations
- Making rounds in various facilities (hospitals, nursing homes, etc.)
- First-assisting in surgery
- Performing minor surgical procedures
- Administering immunizations

An essential part of the PA's job description is working in collaboration with various health care team members, physicians, nurses, medical assistants, surgeons, phlebotomists, and many other allied health care professionals. The scope of practice of a PA is heavily dependent upon the type of practice the PA works in, state regulations, experience, and comfort level of the supervising physician.

Some benefits that PAs enjoy include a flexible schedule, lateral mobility (being able to move from one specialty to another without any formal training), and a high patient satisfaction rate. I've personally worked in five different areas of medicine since becoming a PA in 1994, and I owned a bariatric medicine practice for eight of those years. I hired a supervising physician to sign charts. I had 17 employees, including five PAs, and we saw 90 patients per day.

THE EVOLUTION OF THE PA PROFESSION: FROM PETER THE GREAT TO POSTGRADUATE DEGREES

The PA profession has an amazingly long history. References to various military medical assistants go back as far as 1650 in the Russian army led by Peter the Great. In the World War II era, Dr. Eugene Stead Jr. developed a curriculum model to fast-track the training of physicians in a 3-year time frame.

From 1961 to 1972, the PA concept came more into focus when Dr. Stead established the first PA program at Duke University in 1967. He used much the same model that he had used to train World War II physicians. However, he saw the need for midlevel health practitioners to complement the services and skills of the physicians. The demand was even more apparent in the remote areas of the United States, where the medical profession historically did not reach out to underserved populations. The opening of more PA programs during the ensuing period prompted the development of the PA professional organization, AAPA, in 1968. In 1970, Kaiser Permanente was the first health maintenance organization to employ PAs. And, in 1971, Montefiore Medical Center established the first postgraduate surgical residency program.

The American Medical Association's Committee on Allied Health Education and Accreditation developed training program guidelines in 1971 and implemented the program accreditation process to maintain consistency throughout PA programs. In 1973, the AAPA held its first conference. The first certifying exam was given in 1973, even before the National Commission on Certification of Physician Assistants (NCCPA) became incorporated in 1975.

The NCCPA ensures the public that certified PAs meet established criteria and continue to meet those criteria every 6 years by taking a recertification examination. (As of the time of this writing, the recertification process is now 10 years.) The first recertification exam was in 1981. Also, there has been additional legislation at the state level concerning PA practice and prescriptive privileges. National legislation also addressed PA reimbursement. By 1985, the ranks of PAs had grown to more than 10,000 nationally, prompting the development of *National PA Day* in 1987. By 1988, the AAPA published the first edition of the *Journal of the American Academy of Physician Assistants*, complementing the field's first official journal published in 1977, *Health Practitioner* (later called *Physician Assistant*).

In the 10 years after 1990, misconception and prejudices about PA privileges continued to fall away, allowing for an expanded role for PAs. In addition, discussion and implementation of master's-level programs began to occur, and by 1993, there were 26,400 PAs in existence. By 2002, the number of certified PAs grew to 45,000. The number of PAs grew to 108,717 by 2015, and there are currently (2020) over 148,000 certified PAs in the United States (Figures 1.1 and 1.2).

As of 2021, there are 277 PA programs in the United States.

- 75 Programs with provisional accreditation
- 20 Programs developing—not accredited
- 22 Programs on probation

Figure 1.1. Growth of the PA Profession (1967–2020)

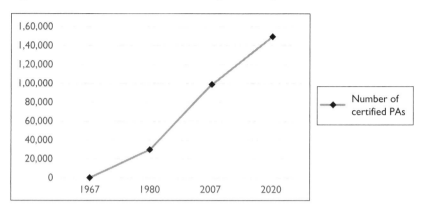

Figure 1.2. Growth of PA Programs (1967–2021)

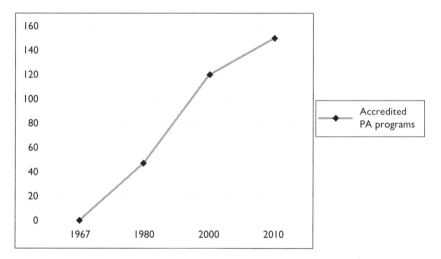

There are also several postgraduate residency programs (Appendix 1) in specialties as diverse as:

- Acute/critical care
- Cardiology
- Cardiothoracic/critical care
- Cardiothoracic surgery
- Child/adolescent psychiatry

- Emergency medicine
- Hematology/oncology
- Hospital medicine
- Neonatology
- Ob-Gyn
- Oncology
- Orthopedic surgery
- Otolaryngology
- Primary care
- Psychology
- Sports medicine
- Surgery
- Surgery/critical care
- Trauma/critical care
- Vascular surgery

The adoption of the PA model in many countries has also resulted in many new PAs. In addition, those internationally trained PAs now represent their home countries at the annual AAPA conference.

How Are PAs Trained?

The length of PA programs varies from 24 to 32 months, depending on whether the program offers a bachelor's degree or a master's degree. Like Quinnipiac University in Connecticut, some programs also provide an Entry-Level Master's Physician Assistant program. The program offers the qualified pre-PA student the opportunity to enter a 4-year pre-professional component and a 27-month professional component. Students can join this program right out of high school.

PA students train in the "medical model," similar to that of most medical schools. In fact, the education process for PAs equates to the first three years of medical school. Many PA programs affiliate with a medical school, and the PA students often share classes with the medical students. The main difference between PA training and physician training is the number of years a physician is required to spend in an internship and residency after the didactic phase of the program.

Students in their first year of a PA program can expect to invest approximately 87 hours per week in the classroom, studying evenings and weekends, and doing some form of volunteer work.

In the second year of PA school, students typically begin clinical rotations. Students work on-site with clinical preceptors at both mandatory and elective clinical rotation sites. Typical mandatory rotations at many programs include:

- Internal medicine
- Family practice
- Emergency medicine
- General surgery
- Pediatrics
- Psychiatry
- Ob-Gyn

You will also have the opportunity to select two or three elective rotations in various specialties and clinical rotation sites. The number of hours you work per week on clinical rotations depends on the specialty and the preceptors. For example, psychiatry may be a 9 to 5 schedule, whereas Ob-Gyn may be over 100 hours per week as it was for me.

During clinical rotations, you will be assigned a preceptor for 6 weeks on average. In the hospital setting, you will typically work with a chief resident. The *team* may consist of other PA students, medical interns, medical residents, and medical students. In the hospital setting, you may have a few patients to follow and *round* on daily. You will complete a history and physical exam, review diagnostic studies, document notes, and report all of your findings to the chief resident and the rest of the team.

In a clinic setting, like family practice, you typically work with an assigned preceptor. I am an *Adjunct Clinical Professor* at Quinnipiac's PA program. I precept students for 6 weeks to accomplish their family practice rotation. In addition, students learn to perform yearly physical exams, wellness visits, and sick visits. First, I bring the student into the room with me, introduce them to the patient, gain permission from the patient to allow the student to perform a history and physical exam. I will then leave the room, and the students report their findings and differential diagnosis to me. Finally, the student will propose a treatment plan, and we will discuss the options. Finally, we go back into the room together to discuss this plan with the patient.

I found that when taking the Physician Assistant National Certification Examination after I graduated, I was able to answer many of the test questions based on my clinical experiences, in addition to my didactic training.

The Future of the PA Profession

To project the future of the PA profession, we must first look at the Association for American Medical Colleges' prediction of a nationwide physician shortage of primary care doctors between "46,000 and 90,000" by 2025.

PAs are likely to fill this gap. According to the Bureau of Labor Statistics (BLS), PAs' job outlook will grow 31% from 2019 to 2029, much faster than the average for all occupations. In addition, as demand for health care services grows, PAs will be needed to provide care to patients.

Salaries for PAs

According to the BLS's Occupational Employment Statistics Survey (2021), the median pay in the United States is $115,390. Many PAs earn over $130,000 per year, and many others earn $200,000 or more. It all depends on your specialty, the number of years of experience, and your negotiating skills.

Making the Case to Choose a Career as a PA versus MD

I often hear this question from PA school applicants, "Should I become a physician assistant or a physician?" Of course, the answer to that question is always a personal one; however, here are six benefits to choosing a career as a PA versus becoming a physician:

1. *PAs spend less time in the classroom*
   Time to obtain a medical license:
   MD: 9–13 years (counting undergraduate degree)
   PA: 6–7 years (including undergraduate degree)
2. *Becoming a PA is very rewarding*
   The work environment for PAs is much more suited to their personality. Where MDs and PAs perform the same duties, PAs have a

greater focus on patient care. PAs don't need to worry about budgets, billing, collections, and bureaucracy.

PAs also get to feel like part of a team. Physicians are independent practitioners (leaders), who often find themselves running a department or practice.

3. *PAs earn an excellent salary*

As mentioned above, the median salary is over $115,390, and many PAs earn much more. According to the BLS, the median salary for a physician is $187,200 per year. Additionally, because it takes about twice as long to become a physician versus a PA, the loan burden is nearly double for a physician versus a PA. This translates to PAs having much more net money in their paychecks.

4. *PAs have flexible hours*

Physicians train to work in one specialty area for their entire career. For example, if a physician becomes a cardiologist, she will stay a cardiologist for the remainder of her career. However, if she decides to change her specialty to gastroenterology, she will need to accomplish a fellowship, which will result in a loss of income.

Once you become a certified physician assistant, you already have the training to work in any medicine or surgery specialty area. That means you can transition from family cardiology to gastroenterology without heading back to the classroom or incurring any loss of revenue.

5. *PAs work shorter, more regular hours*

Physicians not only spend time on patient care, but they must also analyze the practice's revenue and expenditures long after the patients have gone home, and they often work many hours on call.

PAs keep more regular schedules and can choose a position with a lifestyle conducive to their priorities. Then, once the day is over, the PA gets to go home and spend time pursuing outside interests or with their family.

6. *PAs have excellent job prospects*

In today's environment, a PA can probably quit his job in the morning and have a new one by the afternoon. That might be a stretch, but PAs rarely struggle to find work. Busy physicians are always looking for PAs to extend their practices.

As I mentioned above, job growth for PAs is much higher than the national average (31% by 2029) and even faster than physicians. According to the BLS, job growth for physicians and surgeons will increase by 18% over the same period.

Becoming a physician is not the only way to enjoy a fulfilling career in medicine. For these reasons, some people find working as a PA more rewarding.

PAs Scope of Practice

The scope of practice typically includes diagnosing and prescribing treatment plans for patients, ordering labs and diagnostic testing, prescribing medications, referrals to specialists, and much more. However, each state has its scope of practice laws for PAs. The following is a great website to find the scope of practice laws for PAs in any given state may be:

http://www.bartonassociates.com/physician-assistants/physician-assistant-scope-of-practice-laws/

https://beaphysicianassistant.com/blog/optimal-team-practice

What Do PA Programs Look for in a Competitive Applicant?

As you'll discover later on in this book, the PA school admissions committee (ADCOM) members already know the qualities they are looking for in the strongest applicants' way before they even see your Centralized Application Service for Physician Assistants (CASPA) application. Therefore, your goal should be to demonstrate to the committee that you have these qualities. Below is a list of what I feel are the essential qualities you will need to demonstrate to score the highest with the ADCOM. There are also many more specific qualities that I include under each category listed below:

- Passion for the PA profession
- Academic ability and test scores
- Health care experience
- Understanding of the PA profession
- Maturity
- Ability to handle stress

In the following chapters, you will also learn about *soft* skills and *hard* skills.

Okay, so now you know a bit more about the PA profession, and you've made your decision to pursue this exciting career path. In the next chapter, we'll take a look at what you'll need to do to be the most competitive PA school applicant. Then, I will teach you how to go from being a *vanilla* applicant to becoming the *perfect applicant*.

UPDATE FROM THE FOURTH EDITION

Optimal Team Practice (OTP)

In May 2017, the AAPA House of Delegates adopted a new policy that allows its state chapters to seek changes in state laws that, among other things, eliminate the legal requirement for PAs to have a specific relationship with a particular collaborating physician to practice.

There are four components of OTP, which all work toward the same end goals—allowing PAs to practice up to their optimal level of training and removing restrictions that can impede the PAs ability to deliver care.

The four components of OTP include:

1. Team-based practice
2. Elimination of supervisory agreement requirements in laws and regulations
3. Creation of autonomous state boards
4. PA eligibility for direct payment by all public and private insurers

To learn more about OTP, check out the following two websites:
https://beaphysicianassistant.com/blog/optimal-team-practice
https://www.aapa.org/advocacy-central/optimal-team-practice/

CHAPTER 2

What Do PA Programs Look for in a Competitive Applicant?

*G*etting accepted to physician assistant (PA) school is *highly* competitive, and it has been so for several decades. Therefore, you would think that most applicants do their best to meet or exceed all of the minimum requirements to become competitive applicants. I wish this were the case, but after 24 years (to date) of coaching PA school applicants, I can tell you that frequently *is not* the case.

If you frequent the PA Forum (physicianassistantforum.com) as I have, or if you have read the thousands of emails that I have received over the years, you will find that many applicants are looking to get into PA school, skating by with the *minimum* requirements listed on a program's website. These applicants convince themselves that if a PA program requires no medical experience, there is no need to acquire medical experience. They expect, mistakenly, that they will be as competitive as everyone else.

The problem is that over three-quarters of *accepted* PA school applicants come into the application process with prior medical experience (more on this later in the chapter). So although a program doesn't require medical experience, you won't be very competitive without it.

Don't believe me? Let's look at the essential qualities most PA programs look for in the strongest applicants and consider the published data (below) related to *accepted* students. The five important qualities include passion, academic experience, test scores, medical experience, understanding of the PA profession, and maturity.

PASSION

Passion is the rocket fuel that can propel an otherwise-average candidate to the top of the applicant pool. Passion is the burning desire that motivates the perfect applicant to study that extra hour, take that additional chemistry course, repeat classes where they have done poorly, or gain another year of hands-on medical experience *before* applying to PA school. Passion takes the words *I can't* and replaces them with; *I will*. Passion cannot be taught; it must come from deep within.

Unfortunately, too many applicants want to cut corners because of their desire to apply to PA school now! These applicants do not want to do the *necessary work to become competitive applicants,* as demonstrated in the data included in Tables 2.1 to 2.4.

If you truly have the passion for becoming a PA, you will take specific steps and do the work necessary to be the most competitive. Here are ten steps successful PA school applicants will take to become the perfect applicant:

STEP 1: Take an extra year to strengthen their application (if necessary).

STEP 2: Accomplish *all* of the prerequisites needed to become a competitive applicant where they apply.

STEP 3: Find a way to gain another year of medical experience, if required.

STEP 4: Retake extra science courses or those science courses where they did not receive a competitive grade.

STEP 5: Join the American Academy of Physician Assistants (AAPA).

STEP 6: Join their constituent/state chapter of the AAPA.

STEP 7: Find four PAs to shadow.

STEP 8: Do their homework on the programs where they plan to apply. (More on how to do this is provided in the interview chapters; see Chapters 7–9.)

STEP 9: Learn to write a *killer* essay; have it reviewed and edited before submitting it.

STEP 10: Review interview questions and answers, and practice a mock interview before the big day.

Remember, there is no easy way, or shortcut, to get into PA school. You must *do the work* and earn your seat in a program.

A key benefit of having passion is the motivation it provides. For example, on Saturday nights, when you prefer to be out with your friends rather than studying pharmacology or microbiology, your passion will keep you focused. Likewise, on clinical rotations, when you are spending your nights in the on-call room at the hospital, rather than sleeping in your bed, it is your passion for becoming a PA that will make it all seem worthwhile.

Exercise

List five things you've done to demonstrate your passion for becoming a PA. Examples might include shadowing experiences, medical experience, taking additional science courses to raise your Grade Point Average (GPA), making up for a poor grade, becoming a member of the AAPA, and your state/constituent chapter of the AAPA.

1. _____
   _____

2. _____
   _____

3. _____
   _____

4. _____
   _____

5. _____
   _____

Academic Ability and Test Scores

While reviewing your application, the admissions committee (ADCOM) will consider two key factors:

1. Do you have the academic ability to complete a rigorous didactic program?
2. If you complete the program, will you be able to pass your boards?

There is no absolute way to answer these questions with 100% certainty. However, you should be aware of accepted students' average GPA and Graduate Record Examinations (GRE) scores as reported on their websites. Tables 2.1 and 2.2 show first-year class median GPA and GRE numbers.

How do your GPA and GRE scores compare with former, first-year, accepted students? Are you a competitive applicant?

Table 2.1. First-Year Class: Grade Point Averages

GPA Category	M	SD	Median	n(P)
Overall undergraduate:	3.52	0.14	3.52	176
Undergraduate science	3.47	0.16	3.49	163
Centralized Application Service for Physician Assistants (CASPA) biology, chemistry, physics (BCP)	3.42	0.17	3.45	84
Undergraduate non-science	3.54	0.20	3.59	88

Table 2.2. First-Year Class GRE Scores

GRE Scores	M	SD	Median	n(P)
Verbal reasoning	152.2	5.32	153	59
Quantitative reasoning	152	3.68	152	55
Analytical writing	3.9	0.28	4.0	50

Exercise

Fill in the blanks and compare your data to the data above.

Table 2.3. My GPA

GPA Category
Overall undergraduate:
Undergraduate science
CASPA BCP
Undergraduate non-science

Table 2.4. My GRE Scores

GRE Scores
Verbal reasoning:
Quantitative reasoning
Analytical writing

Are you now feeling depressed? Hopeless? Don't worry; the above numbers represent *median* scores, the *midpoint* value. The good news is that ADCOMs will also consider *trends* rather than absolute numbers. For instance, if your GPA is 3.1, but your last ten hard science courses were all A's, you show an upward trend. The committee may consider this when reviewing your application and deciding if you can handle graduate-level science coursework. Of course, I always recommend retaking science classes where you may have done poorly.

Let's look at a hypothetical example of what I'm talking about in Table 2.5, comparing Mary's trend to Bob's.

Table 2.5. Grade Trends

Year in School	Mary		Bob	
Freshman	General chemistry:	D	General chemistry:	A
	Microbiology:	C	Microbiology:	A
Sophomore	Organic chemistry I:	C	Organic chemistry I:	A
	Biochemistry I:	B	Biochemistry I:	B
Junior	Inorganic chemistry:	A	Inorganic chemistry:	C
	Organic chemistry II:	A	Organic chemistry II:	C
Senior	Physical chemistry:	A	Physical chemistry:	C
	Genetics:	A	Genetics:	D

In the above table, we can see that both Mary and Bob have a 3.0 GPA. Mary's trend is upward, and Bob's trend is downward, as evidenced by the above data for each successive year in undergraduate school.

Suppose both Mary and Bob were to take five or six post-graduate science courses or retake the courses where they've done poorly. In that case, they can also demonstrate an upward trend and possibly convince the ADCOM that they can do the work, especially if they have a competitive application otherwise.

Additionally, remember that *median* scores mean that half of the applicant's GPAs are above the median score, and half of the applicant's GPAs are below the median score. So if you're GPA is slightly below the mean GPA for accepted students, don't despair.

Here are some other things the ADCOM will consider.

Number of Credit Hours per Semester

A typical day in PA school requires students to sit in a classroom for 8 to 10 hours per day, perhaps spend an early evening physical examination seminar, and then study for 3 or 4 hours afterward in preparation for a pharmacology exam the next day. This rigorous daily schedule demands excellent time-management skills, as well as the ability to comprehend and assimilate large volumes of scientific material. The only way ADCOMs have to evaluate whether they can make the grade in this area is by reviewing your transcripts. Applicants who carried a full course load, played a sport, and worked part-time will likely make a more favorable impression with the committee than an applicant who took fewer classes and did not participate in any extracurricular activities.

Course Difficulty

The ADCOM will more likely favor an applicant who was a chemistry major with a 3.2 GPA versus an applicant who was a history major with a GPA of 3.4. Remember, the ADCOM is looking for applicants who will thrive while accomplishing graduate-level science coursework.

The Reputation of the College/University

Although the interpretation of GPAs from an Ivy League school versus a State University can be very subjective, I think you would agree that a

3.3 GPA from Harvard would trump a 3.6 GPA from a state school or community college. I only mention this because many applicants will take several classes at a community college and think an "A" is an "A," but it doesn't necessarily work that way.

Life Difficulties and Circumstances

We all experience challenges and difficulties in the course of our lives, some more than others. The ADCOM will consider these challenges when reviewing your application, especially if you have a lower GPA than most. Some significant stressors include divorce, the death of a parent/sibling/spouse, or a severe medical illness. Demonstrate how you've overcome these challenges and became a stronger person. Don't make excuses or expect pity. Being genuine and honest will go a long way toward making your case.

Extracurricular Activities

Your GPA and GRE scores aren't everything when it comes to the admission process. ADCOMs are seeking well-rounded individuals with real-life experiences. I've read thousands of PA school applications. When I see that someone has been in the military, played a sport in college, or even worked for the Peace Corps, I automatically reflect on this person's inherent qualities that will make them a great student and a great PA.

If an applicant has been in the military, I automatically think of the following qualities:

- Discipline
- Attention to detail
- Leadership
- Teamwork

An applicant who played a college-level sport demonstrates:

- The ability to multitask (travel, practice, and perform well in the classroom)
- Teamwork
- Discipline

Someone who worked in the Peace Corps would tend to be:

- Selfless
- Compassionate
- Empathetic

Think about any extracurricular activities that pertain to you, and be sure to mention them in your essay or at your interview.

Standardized Test Scores

Most programs require GRE scores, and the median scores are listed above. However, while on the ADCOM at Yale, I found that test scores did not significantly affect the decision process. If you have a 3.7 GPA in chemistry, 10 years of medical experience, and 3,000 hours of volunteer work, I could care less if your GRE scores are a bit low. Many people don't do well on standardized tests.

My feeling on test scores is strictly my *opinion* and how I weighed them when I was on the ADCOM at Yale. However, you should be aware that a few schools *do* have an absolute requirement for GRE scores. I'm afraid I disagree with this philosophy, but you must consider it if you apply to one of these programs. Thankfully, these programs are the exception and not the rule!

Medical Experience

I've always been amazed by the fact that young students coming right out of college with no prior medical experience definitively know that they want to become physicians and attend medical school. Most applicants accepted to PA school have over 2,000 hours of patient contact experience, which is a tribute to the PA profession. It is also why those applicants with little or no medical experience are far less competitive than those who have accumulated hours.

Unlike applying to medical school, PA school applicants need to gain medical experience before applying. Tables 2.6 to 2.10 list data relative to various types of medical experience and the mean number of hours of medical experience for students accepted into PA programs.

Table 2.6. Medical Experience Statistics for PA School Applicants

Worked in health care before applying to PA school	79%
Worked less than 1 year or not at all in a health care field	27%
Worked more than 9 years in a health care field	10%
Worked less than 1 year or not at all in a health care field with direct patient contact	35%
Previously worked as a medical assistant	17%
Previously worked as an EMT/Paramedic	9%
Worked as a phlebotomist	9%
Worked as an emergency room technician	8%
Worked in medical reception/records	7%
Worked as a nurse	8%
Worked as an athletic trainer	6%
Reported "other" as health care experience	45%

Note: Respondents were permitted to indicate multiple health care fields; thus, the sum of all fields exceeds 100%.

Table 2.7. Average Health Care Experience Hours of Matriculating Students

Health Care Experience	M	SD	Median	n(P)
Patient contact experience	3,100	3,006	2,325	89
Other health care experience	1,014	943	713	30
Other work experience	2,001	1,771	1,500	21
Community service	425	480	270	32
Shadowing	144	204	88	45

Table 2.8. My Health Care Experience Hours

Health Care Experience	# Hours
Patient contact experience	
Other health care experience	
Other work experience	
Community service	
Shadowing	

Exercise

Fill in the blanks to see how you compare with accepted students.

Table 2.9. My Health Care Experience Hours

Health Care Experience	# Hours
Patient contact experience	
Other health care experience	
Other work experience	
Community service	
Shadowing	

Hopefully, you will better understand why I stress the importance of having medical experience and community service before applying to PA school.

Understanding of the PA Profession

The PA profession is growing by leaps and bounds, projected to be one of the top professions for job growth in the future. The salaries are excellent, and the jobs are plentiful. Because of this favorable outlook, some applicants who apply to PA school are just *testing the waters* or throwing their hat in the ring to see if they can pull off getting accepted into this phenomenal career field. Admission committees can usually spot these applicants a mile away. These applicants don't have a thorough understanding of the PA profession because they're not in it for the right reasons. It is imperative to understand the role of the PA and convince the ADCOM that you genuinely want to become a PA for the right reasons.

Therefore, if you plan on applying to PA school, you must do the work and develop a strong understanding of PAs' role in our health care system. You should also know about current events as well as *hot topics* in the news.

The best way to learn about the role of the PA is to shadow PAs. Shadow PAs in various specialties and observe their roles in different clinical settings. Ask a lot of questions and take notes. Become aware of the challenges PAs face daily. Ask the PAs you shadow what they like and don't like about being a PA. Make sure you walk away from these experiences with a thorough understanding of the PA profession.

The best way to stay current with the PA profession and learn about hot topics in the news is to join the AAPA and your state/constituent chapter of the AAPA. You can learn everything you need to know about the PA profession: current events, hot topics, and PA legislation on these websites. Additionally, you will receive a monthly journal (*Journal of the American Academy of Physician Assistant*) and a monthly or quarterly newsletter from your state chapter if you join these organizations.

You will not regret the modest investment it takes to join these organizations, and you will be way ahead of most of the competition if you do so.

Foreign medical graduates (FMGs) receive far more scrutiny than typical applicants. As a result, FMGs must articulate that they have a thorough understanding of the PA profession. In addition, they must convince the ADCOM that they are fully aware of the *profession's dependent nature.*

Some key questions the ADCOM considers concerning FMGs include:

1. Are you going to be able to adapt to the role of a *dependent* practitioner?
2. Are you using PA school as a stepping-stone to gain access to medical school in the United States?

Let's now examine ten common questions that you will likely be asked relative to your understanding of the PA profession:

1. Why do you want to be a PA?
2. What are some of the challenges facing the PA profession?

3. Tell us about some current events relative to the PA profession.
4. What are some hot topics in the news right now concerning PAs?
5. If you could change one thing about the PA profession, what would that be?
6. What is a *dependent* practitioner?
7. How do PAs differ from MDs?
8. What's the difference between a nurse practitioner and a PA?
9. Why don't you want to become a physician?
10. How many PAs have you shadowed?

In the interview chapters, see Chapters 7–9, I cover answers to many of these questions. But, it is your job to do the work and develop a comprehensive understanding of the PA profession through the ways I discussed above.

Maturity

Although maturity doesn't *necessarily* equate to age, it is a fact that the mean age of a first-year PA student is 26 years. However, I have personally interviewed thousands of younger applicants who display a high level of maturity, even at 21. These applicants have a diverse background, a good deal of medical experience, and the ability to present themselves professionally.

Table 2.10. Age-Related Statistics

First-Year Class: Age	M	SD	Median	n(P)
Age of first-year PA student	26.1	2.51	26.0	170
Age of youngest first-year PA student	21.4	1.23	21.0	168
Age of oldest first-year PA student	44.1	7.57	44.0	168

When I do a mock interview with an applicant, I subconsciously ask myself this question: Would I want this person taking care of my child or wife in the emergency room or intensive care unit?

So how does an applicant demonstrate maturity in an interview? Mature applicants exhibit the following traits:

• They know how to be empathetic yet assertive.
• They can handle stress under fire.

- They know when to call for help.
- They exhibit good judgment.
- They can make quick decisions.
- They are self-aware.
- They are self-starters.
- They won't require constant supervision.
- They don't make excuses for their shortcomings.

The best PA school applicants come from diverse backgrounds and possess a variety of life experiences. Some of the most exciting candidates have careers unrelated to health care at the time of the application. However, these applicants have demonstrated PA programs' qualities in the perfect applicant (more on this in the interview chapters; see Chapters 7–9).

Now that you understand the specific traits the ADCOM looks for in solid applicants, let's see if we can develop your personalized plan to achieve this worthy goal.

CHAPTER 3

Your Path to Success: Setting Goals

I believe we all have goals in life, but how many of us have a plan to carry them out? Goals must be specific, have a deadline for achievement, and must be committed to writing to have the best chance of being realized.

At 16, I had two main goals: becoming an entrepreneur and working in medicine. One may think these goals required separate paths; however, I would ultimately achieve both of these goals, as you will see. In this chapter, I hope to help you achieve your dream of becoming a physician assistant (PA), and I will show you exactly how you can develop your personalized plan.

WHY SET GOALS?

Few people ever bother to set realistic goals in life. Most people are what the famous author and motivational speaker, Zig Ziglar, call *wandering generalities* but need to become *meaningful specifics*. The bottom line is that the competition for admission to PA school is fierce. Without a written goal, a plan of action, and the ability to have a razor-like focus, your chances of being accepted to the program of your choice are slim.

The fundamental problem most people have with setting goals is not time; it's a lack of direction. We all have the same 24 hours each day. So why do some people achieve so much, while others who are equally intelligent and capable cannot seem to accomplish anything? Because the former has written, measurable, and realistic goals, they know how to achieve them. From Stephen Covey to Norman Vincent Peale, numerous authors have discussed how to go about setting goals. They both agree: having specific long-term and short-term goals will lead you to become more creative, which will, in turn, add more excitement and fulfillment to your life.

Do you know why 97% of people never really correctly set goals? As Zig Ziglar says, the answer is fear, or *false evidence appearing real.* But what are we afraid of? Some of us are afraid of failure. Some of us fear the competition. Some of us are afraid of success. After all, there is danger in setting goals—we might achieve them! We've all heard the phrase, *be careful what you wish for.*

But I propose there is more danger in not setting goals, especially the risk of wasting your resources. As they say, *a boat in a dry dock rots more quickly than a boat at sea.* So don't waste *your* resources, and write down your goals today!

If I haven't convinced you of the importance of goal setting yet, perhaps this next story will.

In 1953, a study at Yale University polled graduating seniors about how many of them had written goals and a plan of action for carrying them out. Here are the results of that study:

- Three percent had a complete plan.
- Ten percent had taken some steps.
- Eighty-seven percent had set no goals at all and had no plan of action for life after graduation: wandering generalities!

In 1973, 20 years later, the university polled those same seniors again. This time, researchers asked them about their successes in measurable areas: finances, career, and position in life. Not surprisingly, the 3% of graduates, who had set goals and developed a written plan of action to carry them out, had accomplished more than the other 97% combined.

SEVEN-STEP FORMULA FOR SUCCESS

If you utilize the following seven-step formula for success, you too will accomplish *any* worthy goal in life. Follow these simple steps to maximize your chances of getting into the PA school of your choice:

1. Identify the goal.
2. Set a deadline for achievement.

3. List obstacles to overcome.
4. Identify people and organizations that can help you.
5. List the skills and knowledge required to achieve the goal.
6. Develop a plan of action.
7. List the benefits of achieving the goal, and ask yourself: *What's in it for me?*

Now, take out a piece of paper and begin listing your goals. If you do nothing else with this book, you will at least have completed your personalized goal sheet by the end of this chapter. If you need some help getting started, let's look at my personal goal statement from 1992. You'll notice I wrote mine out in paragraph format, but you may write your goals in any form you desire. The point is to get started and get it done; sooner rather than later!

August 15, 1990

By May 1, 1992, I will be accepted into one or all of the following PA programs: Yale, Florida, or Wake Forest (Bowman Gray). To accomplish this goal, I first have to discuss my desire to become a PA with my wife and convince her that this is the right thing for our family. Next, I need to save money to help my wife support our two children and provide food and shelter for the next two years. Finally, I will stay focused and not listen to those who will say; "You're crazy for doing this. Are you having a mid-life crisis? You are thirty-five years old, have a great job, and will have to give that up to go to school for two years."

I will immediately contact the American Academy of Physician Assistants (AAPA) and the Connecticut Academy of Physician Assistants (ConnAPA) to sign up for affiliate membership and find out what resources are available. I will order a copy of the PA Programs Directory (now available online) and begin writing to several schools, focusing on my three top choices. I will contact the president of ConnAPA and get to know him. I will also visit Yale's PA program, meet with Elaine Grant, the program's dean, and maintain contact with her quarterly. I will also correspond with my two top-choice programs quarterly. I will inquire from each program about my strengths and weaknesses and learn what I can do to become a stronger applicant.

I will shadow several PAs who work in the multi-specialty practice where my wife works. In addition, I will attend as many Open Houses as possible to learn more about the program, have discussions with the students, and learn more about the program's culture.

I will take Anatomy & Physiology (I & II) and microbiology courses to fulfill prerequisite requirements. I will achieve no less than an A in each class. I will also begin volunteering at Saint Raphael's hospital emergency room to gain more current patient contact hours. I will also purchase an SAT study guide and prepare myself to score high on the SATs needed to apply to Yale's PA program.

I plan to continue working full-time, save money, and do volunteer work part-time. I will also take the prerequisite classes in the evening. While volunteering in the hospital, I will discuss my goal with as many PAs as possible and learn about the PA profession and the scope of practice in each specialty.

Once I achieve my goal of getting into the PA school of my choice, I will enjoy many benefits: helping people, job satisfaction, a secure future, challenging and stimulating work, prestige, a sense of accomplishment, and earning an excellent salary.

Fast-forward to 2021. I am in my 27th year of clinical practice as a Yale graduate PA. I have worked in five different areas of medicine, including owning my own medical weight loss practice for 8 years. Deciding to become a PA was one of the best choices I have made in my life. I never regretted it for one instant. If I listened to those saboteurs who advised me not to give up my job when I was applying, I would have never experienced the challenges and opportunities I have had as a PA. By the way, the monetary investment paid off significantly.

Exercise

Before completing this chapter, I would like you to write your goal sheet for getting accepted to PA school. The first thing you will need to do before getting started is select at least five programs you want to attend. You can undoubtedly add more programs if you like. Remember that we will discuss selecting programs in the next chapter, so you can always come back to this later.

List your top five PA programs

1. _____

2. _____

3. _____

4. _____

5. _____

[Steps 1 and 2] Identify your goal and set a deadline for achievement

I will be accepted to the _____PA
program by _____, 20_____.

[Step 3] List obstacles to overcome

- _____
- _____
- _____
- _____
- _____
- _____
- _____
- _____
- _____
- _____

[Step 4] Identify people and organizations that can help you

A few examples are listed below to get you started:

1. AJR Associates (Andy Rodican-PA-C @ andrewrodican.com)
2. The American Academy of Physician Assistants (AAPA)
3. State/constituent chapter of the AAPA
4.
5.
6.

[Step 5] List the skills and knowledge required to achieve your goal

a) Gain 1,000 more hours of patient contact

b) Take microbiology and organic chemistry 2

c) _____

d) _____

e) _____

f) _____

g) _____

h) _____

i) _____

j) _____

[Step 6] Develop a plan of action

_____
_____
_____
_____
_____
_____
_____
_____
_____

[Step 7] List the benefits of achieving the goal, and ask yourself: *What's in it for me? What's the payoff?*

A few examples are listed below:

a) Excellent job-growth potential

b) Job satisfaction

c) _____

d) _____

e) _____

f) _____

g) _____

h) _____

i) _____

Now it's time to write out your personalized goal sheet officially. Again, be as specific as possible, laminate the sheet, put it in a place where you will see it, and read it, every day.

Date: _____/_____/_____

_____

_____

_____

_____

_____

_____

_____

_____

_____

_____

_____

_____

_____

_____

_____

_____

_____

_____

_____

_____

_____

_____

_____

_____

_____

_____

_____

_____

_____

_____

_____

_____

_____

IMAGING

Setting goals and committing them to writing is a powerful way to succeed at anything in life. First, however, I want to mention a technique that most professional athletes and successful people worldwide use to magnify their chances of achieving goals. The method is called *imaging.*

The epigraph to this chapter is what first sparked my interest in using imaging as a tool to reach my goals. Let me share with you how I used this technique to help me get accepted to Yale's PA program:

> When I decided to apply to PA school, I immediately developed my goal sheet and incorporated imaging into my daily routine. For example, while visiting the Yale PA program one day, I asked for an envelope with the PA program's logo. I placed that envelope against the side of my television. Next, every day I would work out in my bedroom on an old NordicTrack ski machine. During that entire workout, I would stare at that envelope with the Yale PA school logo and picture myself walking out to my mailbox (we used snail mail at that time), seeing the envelope, opening it, and reading, "Congratulations . . ."
>
> As I did this every day, my heart rate would increase, and my breathing would become rapid and shallow as if I were really walking to the mailbox and seeing the letter inside. I calculated that I used this technique for almost 200 hours before finally receiving my letter of acceptance.

This technique worked for me, and I am confident it will work for you too. Another tool you can use to *supercharge* your motivation and enhance your chances of achieving your goal is to create a *vision board*. I learned about this technique after reading a best-selling 2006 self-help book titled, *The Secret*. Rhonda Byrne wrote this book based on the law of attraction and claims that positive thinking can create life-changing results such as increased happiness, health, and wealth.

In the book, *The Secret*, one of the contributors mentions using a vision board as a tool to fulfill your goals. You make a vision board by taking a blank poster board and placing various pictures, logos, and any visual material that you can see daily to remind yourself of what you want to achieve in life.

For instance, if you want to attend Baylor's PA program, you might add:

- Pictures of the PA school building
- Pictures of PA students in the classroom
- A PA program logo/letterhead
- Pictures of PAs in clinical practice
- Pictures of PA students graduating
- A typed letter (written by yourself) on PA program letterhead reading: *Dear John. Congratulations, you've been accepted into (insert PA program) program's upcoming class...*

You can do this for any/all of the programs where you wish to attend. Looking at these pictures every day will give your subconscious brain the message that this is your chief goal right now, and your subconscious brain will work for you trying to make this happen.

TAKE A PERSONAL INVENTORY

In addition to creating your goal sheet and making a vision board, I recommend reviewing your qualifications and evaluating those areas needing improvement. Going to PA school will be a significant transition, and before you jump in head first, you will need to take a personal inventory. The best way to approach this personal inventory is to evaluate seven specific areas in your life.

I like to use the analogy of spokes on a wheel. If the spokes are all the same size, the wheel will ride smoothly. However, if some of the spokes are short and some are long, you're going to have a bumpy ride.

The purpose of the personal inventory is to balance out your life so that it will run smoothly.

Periodically, evaluate yourself in the following seven areas (see Figure 3.1):

1. *Appearance:* Do I present myself well? Do I need to lose some weight or buy a new pair of shoes before the interview?

2. *Family:* Is my family supportive of my goal? Will this career change cause conflict in my family life? Am I willing to ignore the skeptics and follow my dream unconditionally?

3. *Financial:* Can I afford to attend PA school now? Can I afford *not* to go to PA school now? Will I be able to obtain student loans? Can I save enough money to make the financial burden less stressful?

4. *Social:* Am I a team player? Will I make a good classmate? What do I have to offer? Am I willing to practice medicine as a dependent practitioner?

5. *Spiritual:* Is it morally right to become a PA at this time? Am I choosing this profession for the right reasons? Am I selfish to my family?

6. *Mental:* Do I need to take additional courses or retake some courses? Am I well-read in the PA profession? Will I have too many distractions?

7. *Career:* Do I thoroughly understand why I want to become a PA versus a nurse practitioner or a physician? Do I fully understand the role of a PA?

Figure 3.1. Self-Evaluation

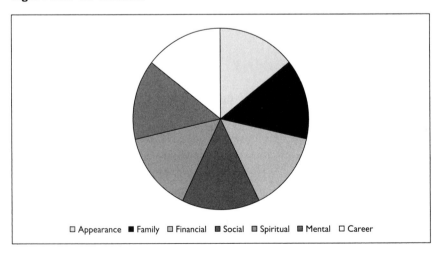

How do your spokes look? Score your answers on a scale from 1 to 5, with 5 being the highest and one lowest. Be honest with yourself. Is your life balanced in these seven areas? Where can you improve? By taking this personal inventory, you will focus on areas where you're deficient and make the necessary changes to reach your goal of becoming a PA.

SET BIG GOALS

I bargained with Life for a Penney,
And Life would pay no more;
However, I begged at evening
When I counted my scanty store.

For Life is a just employer;
He gives you what you ask,
But once you have set the wages,
Why, you must bear the task.

I worked for a menial's hire,
Only to learn, dismayed,
That any wage I had asked of Life,
Life would have willingly paid.

—Jesse B. Rittenhouse

Here's a quick story to drive home the point of setting big goals.

As the story goes, two men were fishing on a pier, one older and one younger. The young man watched as the older man kept reeling in big fish but throwing them back into the water.

Being curious, the young man asked: *Why are you throwing back those big, beautiful fish? Because I only have this small frying pan,* responded the older man, as he held up his tiny skillet.

Without setting big goals, you will never accomplish big things! The old fisherman was a great fisherman, but his skillet—his dream—was too small. So dig down deep into your soul and focus on what you want in life. Then, make a plan and envision yourself accomplishing each task.

TO WHOM DO I SHARE MY GOALS?

We set "give-up" goals designed to let go or get rid of something. For example, if you set a goal to lose 20 pounds of body weight (give-up goal), let everybody in the office, your family, and friends know about it.

In contrast, a "go-up" goal is designed to get you something: a new job, more financial security, an invitation to join a PA program. Share go-up goals only with your closest friends and family members, as they are the ones most likely to support you. When trying to achieve a go-up goal, the last thing you need is to share your plan with a saboteur.

GETTING FOCUSED

I'd like to touch on the power of focus. Just because you've decided to apply to PA school does not mean that *life* stops happening. You will still need to deal with the daily stressors that life throws your way, like finding the time to research schools, completing the Centralized Application Service for Physician Assistants (CASPA) application, working full-time, taking classes in the evening, and managing financial pressures. Some of you may find it overwhelming to deal with these issues and perhaps want to throw in the towel. Don't worry; you're not alone! Everyone feels this way at one point or another during the PA school application process. When you think this way, remember this one saying: *Obstacles are those frightful things we see when we take our eyes off our goal.* Stay focused!

THE TOURNAMENT DRAW TECHNIQUE

Because you will have many items on your "to-do" list, I will share a great technique to get organized and help you accomplish those mini-goals that you will need to complete on your way to your primary goal: getting accepted to PA school.

The number of items you will need to accomplish can seem overwhelming. Therefore, I will share this technique to help you prioritize them by importance.

This technique is patterned after the "March Madness" National Collegiate Athletic Association (NCAA) basketball tournament brackets. At the beginning of the tournament, the NCAA posts the brackets in each division. Those who win continue to progress to the next round.

Eventually, we end up with the "sweet sixteen," the "elite eight," the "final four," and finally, the championship game between the last two teams standing. The winner of the championship game ultimately becomes the NCAA champion.

Table 3.1 patterns this technique. Instead of placing teams in the brackets, you put the items you need to accomplish before selecting a program and completing the CASPA application.

Let's take a look at some of those things you may need to accomplish to apply to PA school:

1. Take the Graduate Record Examinations (GREs)
2. Complete prerequisite microbiology course
3. Shadow one more PA
4. Secure one more person to write a Letter of Recommendation (LOR)
5. Write the essay
6. Gain 500 more hours of medical experience
7. Complete the CASPA application
8. Attend "open houses" at top-choice schools

Now let's put these items into the tournament draw bracket. Just list them on the left side of the bracket in no particular order. Compare each pair of things (#1 with #2) and decide which one is more important, then advance that item to "Round 2." Do the same for items #3 and #4, #5 and #6, and #7 and #8. The point is to keep advancing the essential items to Round 2, then repeat the comparisons until you have a "winner," or the priority you will need to accomplish on your "to-do" list.

I will use eight items in this example, but this technique will work for 16 items, 24 items, or however many you have.

So, let's look at the hypothetical list above and place them into Round 1 of the "Tournament Draw Technique" (Table 3.1).

Here is my rationale for making my choices; your choices certainly may be different. I compared #1 with #2 in Round 1 and decided it was more important to complete the prerequisite microbiology class before taking the GRE. Without the microbiology class, I would not meet all of the program's prerequisites, and I would be ineligible to apply. But, of course, I could always take the GREs later, even concurrently with the microbiology course. The microbiology class, therefore, moves on to Round 2.

Then, I compared #3 with #4 in Round 1, and I decided it is more important to find another PA to shadow before securing another person to write my letter of recommendation. Although both may be equally

Table 3.1. The Tournament Draw Technique Format

Round 1	Round 2	Round 3	Winner
1. Take GREs	Microbiology	Microbiology	Microbiology
2. Take microbiology			
3. Shadow PA	Shadow		
4. LOR			
5. Write essay	Medical experience	Medical experience	
6. Medical experience			
7. Complete CASPA	Attend open house		
8. Attend open house			

important, I believe it will be harder to find a PA to shadow and accumulate hours with that person than securing another person to write my letter of recommendation. I may even be able to have the PA I shadow write a LOR for me. So, shadowing another PA moves on to Round 2.

Next, I compared #5 with #6 in Round 1, and I decided that I need to gain 500 more hours of medical experience to be the most competitive. I could write the essay while accumulating those hours. Therefore, gaining 500 hours of medical experience moves on to Round 2.

Finally, I compared #7 with #8 in Round 1 and decided it would be better to attend the program's open house before accomplishing the CASPA application. I will probably learn a lot about the program at the open house and have an opportunity to meet with students of the program. In addition, the information I learn at the open house will be beneficial to me when writing my essay and answering questions at the interview. Therefore, attending the open house moves on to Round 2.

The process continues by deciding which items move on to the third round and ultimately the winner. In the above example, taking the prerequisite microbiology course is the winner and my number one priority. I can now work backward (Round 3 to Round 1) and continue to accomplish my currently listed preferences in each bracket. For instance, my next goal would be to go back to Round 3 and realize my next goal is to gain 500 hours of additional medical experience. I could also do this part-time while completing the microbiology course. Keep moving backward in the rounds until you are finished. Okay, so now that you've joined the top 3% of achievers by writing down your goals, it's time to look at the multitude of PA programs and decide which programs will be the best "fit" for your qualifications. Choosing programs will be an exciting process, but you must do your homework!

See Appendix 2 for a blank Tournament Draw Technique format that you can accomplish using your to-do list. Remember, you can expand the list, and the chart, to add additional items.

[CHAPTER 4]

Selecting a PA Program

The excitement is starting to build. You've committed to applying to physician assistant (PA) school, you have a written goal, and your next task is to select the program(s) you want to attend. At the time of this writing, there are over 270 programs. You may be a bit overwhelmed at this point, but I want you to realize that you should have a common denominator for all programs you select. So, ask yourself, why am I applying to these particular programs versus any other programs?

One applicant I worked with in the past told me she was asked the following question at her interview:

> Provide us with a list of all the schools you've applied to, why you applied there, which are your top schools and why, where you received interviews, and which is your first choice?

Wow, what a question! Not every program will ask you this question, but you should at least be prepared to answer your rationale for applying to the programs you've chosen.

A FEW QUESTIONS TO CONSIDER BEFORE SELECTING YOUR PROGRAM(S)

1. Is the program accredited by the Accreditation Review Commission on Education for the Physician Assistant (ARC-PA?)

ARC-PA is the accrediting agency that defines PA education standards and evaluates PA educational programs within the territorial United States to ensure compliance with those standards.

The very first criteria you should look for in a PA program you're considering is its accreditation status. The accreditation status of a PA program is listed as follows:

a. Continuing accreditation

A program with a continuing accreditation status is an established program in compliance with the standards of accreditation.

b. Provisional accreditation

Provisional accreditation status is granted for a limited period to a new program demonstrating its preparedness to initiate a program per the standards.

c. Probationary accreditation

Probational accreditation is a temporary status for programs that do not meet current standards and threaten students' satisfactory educational experience.

d. Developing-not accredited

Programs that are working toward accreditation but have not yet passed the ARC-PA accreditation review. There is no guarantee that the program will be accredited.

You can find a current list of the accreditation status of every program on the Physician Assistant Education Association (PAEA) website at: *directory.paeaonline.org/programs/1019*.

2. What is the program's first-time pass/fail rate on the Physician Assistant National Certification Examination (PANCE)?

To become a certified physician assistant (PA-C) after graduating from a PA school, you must pass the PANCE. If you fail the PANCE, you cannot work as a PA; it's that simple.

So, when looking at programs to apply to, I strongly recommend that you consider the program's first-time pass/fail rate on the boards, as well as the 5-year PNCE rates. The average 5-year, first-time pass/fail rates nationally are currently at 94% for all programs.

However, as you will see in Appendix 3, PA programs' first-time pass/fail rates currently range from 69% to 100%. Which program would you prefer to attend? A PANCE rate of 69% means that three out of ten students who've graduated from that program failed the PANCE (first-time). After accreditation status, I would consider high PANCE rates as my second criteria. What a shame it would be to invest 2 years of your time in a program, and possibly over $100,000 for tuition, and not be able to pass your boards and become a PA-C! (See PANCE RATES Appendix 3.)

A word of caution, make sure you look at the *first-time* PANCE rates and not the overall PANCE rates. The National Commission on Certification of Physician Assistants (NCCPA) publishes each program's PANCE rates on each program's website.

3. When did the program begin: longevity of the program?

You may be asking yourself, why is the longevity of the program so important? Won't I have a better chance of getting into a new program?

Let's consider the first question: why is longevity so important? The longevity of the program is essential for a couple of reasons:

- *Track record*: A well-established program typically has (but not always) a winning formula that works to educate students and prepare them to pass the PANCE.
- *Established clinical rotation sites*: It could take several years for a program to rule in or rule out clinical rotation sites that provide the best opportunities for their PA students to learn and have a chance to participate in the care of patients. For example, if you are on a team with interns, residents, and PA students on a surgical rotation, you may be *low man on the totem pole* when it comes to scrubbing in on a surgical procedure in the operating room. Some surgeons may feel an obligation to train the interns and residents first and delegate you to the role of an observer.

Instead of being the *first assistant* on a procedure, you may be the *third assistant,* relegated to holding retractors for the entire case. As a result, you may not be able to see the surgical field. You will not be able to see the anatomy, and you may not practice your suturing skills.

It takes a few years for a program to weed out these rotations based on the student's feedback about that particular rotation.

I found that clinical rotations play a significant role in how well you do on the PANCE. In your didactic training, you are typically memorizing material. In contrast, you may remember answers to a PANCE question in the clinical rotations because you took care of a patient who had the diagnosis discussed in the question. For instance, you may be asked about the medication to treat HIV. You will remember that medication because you took care of patients with HIV in your internal medicine rotation and had to review their medication list every day.

4. *Is the program affiliated with a medical school?* Programs affiliated with medical schools typically have a lot more resources available to them than free-standing programs. In many cases, you will take classes in conjunction with the medical students. Medical schools affiliated with hospitals provide access to the medical school library and many other amenities not afforded to a free-standing program. Additionally, medical schools almost always have cadaver labs, allowing you to learn anatomy on an actual human body versus plastic models or in a simulation lab.

5. *Does the program have a cadaver lab?* As mentioned above, learning anatomy on a cadaver is much more interesting than learning anatomy from slides or plastic models. I believe learning anatomy on a cadaver will make you a better clinician. For example, you get to see the sciatic nerve and understand why we give intramuscular injections to the buttocks to avoid this colossal nerve. You will appreciate why educating your patients with sciatica is essential to avoid placing their wallet in back pockets because of its pressure on the nerve. You will have the opportunity to see and touch the great vessels of the heart, heart valves, and its four chambers to better understand how this miraculous pump works to feed blood to the body.

   You will see and feel the *brachial plexus*, a massive bundle of nerves that run under the armpit. You will understand why we advise patients to keep the cushions of crutches against the side of the chest and not in the armpit to avoid crushing the brachial plexus. I might not have appreciated that visual on a plastic model or a slide.

   Dissecting a human cadaver is a fantastic experience and a great teaching tool.

6. *Where is the program located?* If financial or family circumstances limit your ability to travel, you will probably want to apply to programs within your geographical area. Just keep in mind, some out-of-state programs may be a better fit for your background and your preferences in a program.

7. *Is it a master's program?* In the past 27 years of PA practice, I can honestly say that I've never observed a prospective job applicant accepted or rejected solely based on having a master's degree versus a bachelor's degree. There are so many job opportunities available that the only letters you need after your name are PA-C.

There are a couple of exceptions to this rule; if you want to teach at a PA program or if you want to do research, you will need a master's degree to do both.

After completing a rigorous PA program, I certainly believe that we all probably meet or exceed the requirements for a master's degree. The trend has changed from most PA programs offering bachelor's degrees to most PA programs now offering master's degrees.

In summary, I don't think it matters whether you earn a master's degree or not. I received a graduate certificate at Yale, and not having a master's degree never affected my clinical skills, job prospects, or the ability to open my practice.

8. *Who teaches the classes in the didactic phase of the program?* Many of you may not have thought about this question or don't see how it matters. If a program's first-time PANCE rates are 96%, who cares? However, I believe that you should be familiar with who will provide your didactic training and the differences among the various choices of educators. Here is a nonjudgmental list of options:

   a) *Fellows*: *Fellows* are physicians who've completed their residency and are now investing two or more years learning a specialty like cardiology, dermatology, general surgery, and so on.

   In my opinion, who is better to teach a class in cardiology than a cardiology fellow, someone who is highly motivated and up-to-date on the most current information in the field. Additionally, since fellows are literally at the beginning of their specialized training, they are highly motivated individuals, passionate about their specialty, and less likely to suffer from "burnout."

   b) *Physicians*: Many programs have local physicians who work in the community, or an affiliated medical school, lecture students in their specialty area. The benefit of having physicians teach classes in the didactic phase is that the student will benefit from that physician's many years of clinical experience.

c) *Researchers*: Researchers are probably better able to teach physiology rather than clinical medicine. These are the guys that will present elaborate charts and graphs and discuss the results of various clinical trials related to their field. These will be very scholarly presentations, and they may keep you up late at night trying to digest the information in the lecture.

d) *Physician assistants*: Many programs utilize PAs from the program or the community to teach classes. One obvious benefit of having PAs teach is the fact that they can relate better to your situation. However, one negative is that these PAs might not have experience in the specialty course. Therefore, they may be assigned classes to teach that are not in their specialty area.

9. *How much is the tuition?* In other words, consider how much debt you will be in after you graduate. Of course, tuition varies significantly for each program, and I would certainly evaluate the *pros* and *cons before* you apply.

10. *How much is housing, parking, and the average cost of living in the community?* These costs can add up.

So, if you're asked, "Why have you chosen our program?, you're now armed with a wealth of information to draw upon when providing your answer.

ARE YOU A *GOOD* FIT?

Another essential question you should ask yourself when selecting PA programs is: "Am I a good fit for this program?" What do I mean by this? As you'll see in the interview chapters, PA programs already know the qualities they're looking for in applicants they accept to their program. Your job is to determine these qualities and demonstrate that you have them; you're a good fit. For instance, if a program's website states that they prefer to select in-state applicants and you're not from that state, your odds of getting accepted might not be as favorable as someone from that state. Therefore, you wouldn't necessarily be a good fit for that program.

Additionally, suppose a program's mission statement mentions a *solid commitment to community service*. If you haven't done much community service in the past, you might not be a good fit for that program. I can't stress this enough; it is vital to do your homework before applying to a PA program. It's best to be able to *demonstrate* that you have the qualities the program is seeking. For example, suppose the program values diversity. In that case, you will have a better chance of acceptance if you have a history of working with diverse populations, rather than simply saying you recognize that they value diversity.

If a program has an absolute requirement of a 3.5 science Grade Point Average (GPA) and your science GPA is 3.3, you may not be the best fit for that program.

Please don't get too worried; however, many programs are more liberal regarding absolute requirements.

A NOTE ABOUT *RANKING* PA PROGRAMS

US News & World Report (US News) has historically ranked PA programs. The rankings are typically updated and published every year. *US News* ranks PA programs based on a *subjective* survey of PA school faculty and administration. In my opinion, many PA school applicants, PA students, and PA faculty rely on this report as a valid indicator of a program's success. *US News & World Report* has been publishing results for the top PA programs since 1998.

In an article titled, "A Novel Approach to Ranking Physician Assistant Programs," by James Van Rhee, MS, PA-C and Michael J. Davanzo, MMS, PA-C (*The Journal of Physician Assistant Education*, 2010, vol. 21, no. 4), the author proposed a new approach to ranking PA programs. He based this approach on *objective* data.

PA program directors from 126 accredited PA programs (at the time) identified indicators in a new ranking system for PA programs. The four criteria they agreed upon were:

1. Each program's current ARC-PA accreditation length
2. Student-to-faculty ratio
3. Percentage of faculty with doctoral degrees
4. Most recent 5-year average PANCE rates

If you look at Table 4.1, you can see that in 2007, the new ranking system and the *US News & World Report* ranking systems were pretty different. For example, the University of Wisconsin-La Crosse ranks number one in the new system but doesn't rank in the top 20 in the *US News* system. On the other hand, Duke University ranks number two in the *US News & World Report* ranking system, but not in the top 20 in the new ranking system.

Table 4.1. Comparison of New Ranking and *US News* Ranking

Rank	New Ranking System	Rank	*US News* Ranking 2007
1	University of Wisconsin-La Crosse	1	University of Iowa
2	Oregon Health & Science	2	Duke University
3	University of Iowa	3	Emory University
4	Central Michigan University	4	George Washington University
5	University of TX SW Medical Center	4	University of TX SW Medical Center
6	University of Nebraska	7	University of Utah
7	Rutgers (UMDNJ)	8	University of Washington
8	University of Oklahoma—OKC	9	University of Colorado
9	Quinnipiac University	9	Baylor College of Medicine
9	Emory University	11	Oregon Health & Science
11	DeSales University	11	Interservice PA Program
12	Duquesne University	11	SUNY-Stony Brook University
12	Yale University	14	University of TX Medical Branch Galveston
14	Baylor College of Medicine	14	University of Nebraska

Table 4.1. Comparison of New Ranking and *US News* Ranking (*Continued*)

Rank	New Ranking System	Rank	*US News* Ranking 2007
14	Augsburg College	14	Quinnipiac University
16	University of TX Medical Branch Galveston	17	Rosalind Franklin University
17	SUNY-Stony Brook University	17	Rutgers (UMDNJ)
18	Northeastern University	17	Northeastern University
19	Saint Francis University (PA)	17	Saint Louis University
20	Wayne State University	21	University of TX Health Center San Antonio
20	Philadelphia University	21	Saint Francis University (PA)

So what does this mean to you, the PA school applicant, during your selection process? In my opinion, it means that you have to do your homework and look at the four criteria listed above versus taking the *US News & World Report* data as an absolute indicator of the best PA programs.

I'm a big believer in reviewing a program's first-time PANCE rates to assess the quality of that program. If the program's PANCE rates are high (94% and above), it means they're doing an adequate job of preparing students to pass the boards and ultimately become eligible to practice as a PA. I don't care how prestigious a PA program may be or how high *US News & World Report* ranks a program. If you invest two or more years of your time and possibly $150,000 or more in your education, you'll want to be sure that you will be able to pass your boards once you graduate. If you don't pass your boards, you can't work as a certified PA!

Table 4.2 provides you with a list of PANCE rates of the programs ranked in the top 20 for both ranking systems in 2007. Notice that the University of Wisconsin-La Crosse has a 100% 5-year PANCE rate and ranks as the number one program in the new ranking system.

However, Wisconsin-La Crosse doesn't even show up on the *US News & World* Report ranking system. But the University of Washington, with an 86% 5-year PANCE rate, is number seven on the *US News* list. (https://www.usnews.com/best-graduate-schools/top-health-schools/ physician-assistant-rankings)

Table 4.2. Comparison of the 5-Year, First-Time Pass/Fail Rates of PA Programs in Both Ranking Systems

New Ranking System (2016)	5-Year PANCE Rate (%)	US News Ranking (2007)	Rank (%)
University of Wisconsin-La Crosse	100	University of Iowa	100
Oregon Health & Science	98	Duke University	96
University of Iowa	100	Emory University	95
Central Michigan University	96	George Washington University	94
University of TX SW Medical Center	100	University of TX SW Medical Center	100
University of Nebraska	98	University of Utah	93
Rutgers (UMDNJ)	97	University of Washington	86
University of Oklahoma—OKC	97	University of Colorado	98
Quinnipiac University	98	Baylor College of Medicine	97
Emory University	95	Oregon Health & Science	98
DeSales University	100	Interservice PA Program	97
Duquesne University	92	SUNY-Stony Brook University	97

Table 4.2. Comparison of the 5-Year, First-Time Pass/Fail Rates of PA Programs in Both Ranking Systems (*Continued*)

New Ranking System (2016)	5-Year PANCE Rate (%)	*US News* Ranking (2007)	Rank (%)
Yale University	98	University of TX Medical Branch-Galveston	98
Baylor College of Medicine	97	University of Nebraska	98
Augsburg College	99	Quinnipiac University	98
University of TX Medical Branch-Galveston	98	Rosalind Franklin University	95
SUNY-Stony Brook University	97	Rutgers (UMDNJ)	97
Northeastern University	97	Northeastern University	97
Saint Francis University-Pennsylvania	96	Saint Louis University	99
Wayne State University	96	University of TX Health Center-San Antonio	95
Philadelphia University	94	Saint Francis University-Pennsylvania	96

There were 19 PA programs with 100% first-time pass/fail rates on the PANCE, yet only three of those programs made the *US News* top 20 lists.

FINAL THOUGHTS ON SELECTING A PA PROGRAM

I would be remiss if I did not mention this final thought that is so important to consider when selecting a PA program. I will cover this information in greater detail in Chapter 7, but I cannot stress this concept enough.

When selecting a PA program, you will need to do your homework and select programs that are a good *fit* for your qualifications. As you will learn in Chapter 7, *It's not about you; it's about them!* Do you have the qualities the PA program prefers in accepted students?

PA programs already know what qualities they're looking for in candidates *before* reviewing your application and before your interview. It is your job to show them that you possess these qualities and demonstrate them in your essay and interview.

So when you begin researching programs, you must understand what qualities each program is looking for in the perfect applicant. To reiterate, if you want to apply to a program that values candidates who've worked in *underserved areas,* and you have never done so, you won't satisfy their needs compared to an applicant who's worked in soup kitchens or has gone on missions to impoverished countries. I'm not saying you won't have a chance of getting accepted, but you won't be as strong an applicant as those who have done so.

Let's say you want to apply to Duke's PA program. If you do your homework, you will see that Duke's website, *What We Look for in an Applicant,* lists the following specific qualities they are seeking:

- Cultural diversity
- Applicants who are underrepresented in the PA profession
- A heart for service
- Volunteerism
- Military service
- North Carolina residents from geographically underserved areas such as Area Health Education Centers (AHEC)
- Years of experience in the healthcare field

These qualities are in addition to the rigorous academic, patient contact hours, and Graduate Record Examination scores they require.

I will cover this area in greater detail in the interview chapters (see Chapters 7–9), but remember that it is your job to research each program you will be applying to and find out what qualities they value most. Then, ask yourself, "Can I *demonstrate* these qualities?" If not, you may want to look for programs where you will be a better fit or choose to get more experience in these areas before you apply.

Okay, now that you've selected your top choice programs, let's discuss the Centralized Application Service for Physician Assistants (CASPA) application process in this next chapter.

CHAPTER 5

The Application Process: The Centralized Application Service for Physician Assistants (CASPA) (caspaonline.org)

You're now ready to begin the application process for physician assistant (PA) school. You feel inspired and motivated. Then you look at the CASPA application, and perhaps you become intimidated by the seemingly complex process. Don't worry; you're not alone. The most extensive advice I can give you is:

- Apply early
- Follow instructions
- Pay strict attention to detail
- Read the FAQ section

You'll find the answers to 99% of all your questions on the FAQ page. So, don't be lazy; find the topic where you may have questions and read the entire section. Also, be sure to start with the *Before You Create an Application* section first.

I will also cover some of the most common CASPA FAQs at the end of this chapter.

BACKGROUND ON THE CASPA APPLICATION

Before 2001, PA school applicants had to accomplish separate applications for each program. Applicants had to complete a lot of paperwork, write more than one essay, and pay a fee for every application. The cost alone certainly limited many applicants from applying to multiple programs.

In 2001, the Physician Assistant Education Association (PAEA) began using CASPA. This service allows applicants to complete a single online application and send the completed application to any PA program the applicant designates. In 2021 (currently), the cost for a CASPA application is $179 for the first application and $55 for each additional program that utilizes CASPA.

Keep in mind that not all PA programs utilize the CASPA application at this time (about 10%), and if you apply to one—or more—of these programs, you will have to complete a separate application and pay the appropriate fees.

You may also have to accomplish *supplemental* applications for some programs. More on this later in the chapter. You will find information on the CASPA application process at https://caspa.liaisoncas.com/applicant-ux/#/login

BENEFITS OF THE CASPA APPLICATION

Since CASPA online applications became available in 2001, I've coached thousands of applicants and reviewed hundreds of CASPA applications. I've listened to the feedback from these applicants concerning the CASPA application process and why they like using this service. Here are some of the benefits you'll appreciate most:

1. The ability to apply to multiple programs using a single online application.
2. The checklist and instructions provided on the CASPA website simplify the process of accomplishing the application.
3. Data only has to be entered once, such as transcripts, letters of recommendation (LOR), health care experience, and demographic data.
4. The ability to access the CASPA application from any computer, update information, and save it right up until it's submitted for final verification.

Apply Early

The CASPA application cycle runs from April every year until the following March. I strongly recommend starting your application ASAP, even if you don't have everything you need to complete it. Many programs utilize a *rolling admissions* format; they evaluate and process applications on a first-come, first-served basis. They either select the applicant for an interview on the spot or reject the applicant. Once they meet their quota for interviewees, the process is closed. You can find a current list of programs that utilize rolling admissions in Appendix 4.

Follow Instructions

Failure to follow instructions can be a fatal move on your part. The CASPA application is only verified once you provide *all* the requested information. I will give you some tips later in this chapter but read the *Before You Create An Application* section on the CASPA website when all else fails.

Pay Strict Attention to Detail

Paying strict attention to detail is an important quality you will need to have as a good clinician. I know that you will be excited to get the ball rolling and complete your application as soon as possible; however, if you rush through the process and don't pay strict attention to every detail, you will undoubtedly regret it later.

Let me give you a personal example of the importance of paying strict attention to detail:

> After graduating from college in 1984, I decided to become an air force officer. So I signed up at the recruiting station, and before I knew it, I was on my way to San Antonio, Texas, to begin Officer Training School (OTS).
>
> OTS is a highly intense twelve-week program. To be a competent officer, you must exhibit many qualities required to be an effective leader. One of those qualities is the ability to pay strict attention to detail.
>
> We had to accomplish several *measurements* to show we have what it takes to become an officer from the first day. If you fail three measurements during the 12 weeks of training, you're out of OTS and get sent to the enlisted ranks. The measurements included: physical requirements, academic requirements, and military bearing requirements.
>
> In the first week of training, we had to accomplish our first requirement: a simple multiple-choice test. The instructor told us we had only five minutes to complete the test. Having to answer 50 questions in 5 minutes, or ten questions per minute, made me extremely anxious. I couldn't flunk my first measurement!
>
> The proctor handed out the exam and advised us that we could not pick up our pencils until he said "Begin," and we had to drop our pencils when he said, "Stop" immediately. My heart started racing.
>
> The proctor then said, "Begin!" I looked down at the paper and noticed a tiny paragraph at the top of the page. I then glanced at the rest of the exam and read some seemingly simple, basic questions. Piece of cake, I thought. However, this almost seemed too easy.
>
> To complete this measurement on time, I skipped the first paragraph and began answering the questions immediately. I was a bit surprised at how easy the questions were, and I began to relax.
>
> All of a sudden, I got this pit in my stomach. Something was wrong. I briefly looked up and discovered many of the other candidates had their pencils on the table and weren't answering the questions. Odd, I thought. I then refocused on the test and completed the exam well in advance of the time limit.
>
> The proctor said, "Stop," and I immediately dropped my pencil. I was thrilled with my performance and felt very relaxed.
>
> Then the proctor said those dreadful words that I can still hear today: "If you answered *any* of these questions, you failed this measurement." My heart sank; what does he mean? He then went on to tell us all to read that first paragraph I decided to skip. It clearly stated, *do not pick up your pencil and do not answer any of these questions.*

> I failed to pay strict attention to detail, and I bombed my first measurement. Two more failures, and I was out. However, I learned my lesson and did not flunk another measurement during those 12 weeks.

The take-home message here is to pay strict attention to detail on your CASPA application. Read everything! Take the process step-by-step, and you'll get through it. Thousands of applicants have done it before you and know that you can do it too.

Read the FAQ Section

I probably could have started and ended this entire chapter with the above heading. But, trust me, everything you need to know is on the CASPA website, especially the FAQ section. CASPA lays it out in perfect order. All you have to do is follow directions. Enough said!

Seven Practical Tips for Completing the CASPA Application

I'm going to provide you with seven tips to make the CASPA application process a little easier:

1. Follow instructions. As mentioned already, take the application process step-by-step, follow all of the instructions, and pay strict attention to detail.
2. List five names of those people you plan to ask for a LOR, and be sure to give them a *heads up* about the format and time requirement. They need to understand how important it is to accomplish their letters on time. (I will provide a complete section on the LOR later.)
3. Be sure to request your transcripts early and have them sent directly to *you.*

   The sooner you receive your transcripts, the sooner you can accomplish the coursework section of the application.
4. Do not exceed the 5000-character limit on your essay. If you do, the remaining characters will not get entered. Your essay will be incomplete, showing your complete lack of attention to detail.
5. Ensure that you write down the application deadlines for each program you are applying to and adhere to those deadlines. If the program utilizes rolling admissions, submit your application the day the CASPA cycle opens.

6. Do your homework. Visit the websites of all the programs you've chosen, and be sure that you meet or exceed all of the requirements and prerequisites. Some programs won't even look at your application if you haven't met their needs. Remember, they may get 1,000 applications, and most of those applicants will have all of the requirements; why would they choose you if *you* don't meet their criteria?

7. Apply early. Register as soon as you decide to apply to PA school, and try to get your CASPA application accomplished several weeks before each programs' application deadline, primarily if they utilize rolling admissions (Appendix 4). Start acquiring the following information that you will need to accomplish the application:

    a) A complete accounting of your health care experience, including the number of hours accumulated (at the time of application) and dates of employment. Document dates and duties of all of your volunteer experiences as well as your shadowing experiences.

    b) Obtain a personal copy of required test scores.

    c) Collect copies of any certificates you may have earned, including awards, certifications (Emergency Medical Technician, Advanced Cardiac Life Support), specialized training.

    d) Obtain written transcripts ASAP.

    e) Decide whom you will choose to write your LOR. (See Chapter 6 for more details.)

CASPA APPLICATION STATUS AND NOTIFICATIONS

A word of caution regarding notifications from CASPA: they will *not* email you if you have any incomplete data in your file. You must be proactive and frequently check the status of your application regularly. The last thing you need to discover a week before a deadline is that one of your referees failed to submit her letter on time.

To check the status of your application, open your application on the CASPA website, click on *Manage My Programs*, then click on *Program Status*. The following is a list of statuses you may find:

1. In Progress
2. Received—Awaiting Materials
3. Materials Received—Verifying

4. Complete Date
5. Complete Date Currently Being Verified
6. Undelivered
7. Verified

Why Is My CASPA GPA Different from the One on My Transcripts?

Many applicants become bewildered when they notice discrepancies between their Grade Point Average (GPA) as calculated on their college transcript(s) and their GPA as calculated on the CASPA application. Why is this? If you look at the FAQ page on CASPA's website, you will see that there are four reasons for this:

1. CASPA does not recognize individual schools' forgiveness or grade replacement policies regarding repeated courses.
2. CASPAs numeric scale for letter grades may differ from the one used at the institutions you attended (see Table 5.1).
3. CASPA calculates all GPAs in semester hours. Thus, if you completed quarter hours, CASPA will convert those grades to semester hours; 1.0 quarter-hour = 0.667 semester hours.
4. CASPA breaks down your GPA by college level (freshman, sopho-more, etc.). So, if you attended multiple colleges and took freshman classes, they will all fall under your freshman GPA.

When calculating your GPA, CASPA utilizes:

• Quality Points (QP)
• The letter grade of each course
• The semester hours for each course
• Cumulative attempted hours for all courses

The formula is as follows:

Number of Credit Hours × Letter Grade = Quality Points
Number of Quality Points/Total Credit Hours = Calculated GPA

Please note that a "W" counts the same as an "F" according to CASPA calculations. You can manually calculate these numbers, or you can go to (https://www.thepaplatform.com/pa-school-gpa-calculator). You can enter your grades and credit hours and obtain your CASPA GPA.

Table 5.1. CASPA Letter Grade Values

Transcript	Letter Grade	Value
A+	A	4.0
A	A	4.0
A–	A–	3.7
AB	AB	3.5
B+	B+	3.3
B	B	3.0
B-	B-	2.7
BC	BC	2.5
C+	C+	2.3
C	C	2.0
CD	CD	1.5
D+	D+	1.3
D-	D-	0.7
E	F	0.0
F	F	0.0
WF	F	0.0

LETTERS OF RECOMMENDATION (LOR)

As part of the CASPA application process, you need to provide at least three LOR supporting your application. Be sure to pay strict attention to detail relevant to each school's specific requirements for whom they want as referees. For example, some programs may allow you to choose from your references. Others may specify that you need letters from a *PA, a physician, and a former supervisor.*

When considering candidates to provide your LOR, I advise that you ask at least one PA to write it (unless otherwise specified). After all, who is better to write about the qualities you possess to become a good PA than a PA? Additionally, the PA profession consists of a tight-knit and protective group of health care professionals. We want to be sure that if we recommend an applicant for PA school, that person is a high-quality applicant. So, an LOR from a PA probably carries the most weight with respect to any other choices. Unfortunately, many applicants fail to realize the importance of securing an LOR from a PA. For example, many applicants will write about shadowing a PA in their essay but fail to include a recommendation letter from that person in their CASPA application.

Another huge mistake some PA school applicants make when selecting individuals to write their LOR is to assume the more prominent the name or status of the referrer (the *big shot*), the more weight the LOR will carry. Nothing could be further from the truth!

Let me give you an example of what I mean. Some applicants will ask a *big shot* to write an LOR for them. The *big shot* agrees, and all is well. The applicants feel confident the LOR from this person is going to boost their chances.

Then 1 week before the school's deadline, the applicant realizes his CASPA application is not verified yet. He's still missing one LOR. Guess whose letter is missing? That's right, the *big shot*. Now what? The *big shot* is typically unavailable to take your phone calls; she is not responding to your emails, and because she is a *big shot*, you are afraid of being too pushy.

Be sure you will feel comfortable contacting your referees if they are cutting it close to the deadline and give them a little push to get the LOR submitted as soon as possible.

What Makes an Effective Letter of Recommendation?

I recommend that the writer of your LOR comment on the following areas:

- Academic performance
- Interpersonal skills
- Maturity
- Adaptability and flexibility

- Motivation for a career as a PA
- Ability to work collaboratively with others
- Strengths relative to a career as a PA

A strong LOR also includes four specific features:

1. It shows that the writer genuinely knows the individual and can comment about the applicant's qualifications.
2. It shows that the writer knows enough about the applicant and can make comparative judgments about the applicant's intellectual, academic, and professional abilities relative to others in a similar role.
3. It provides supporting details to make the statement believable.
4. It is short yet concise and sincere.

Who Should Write Your Letter of Recommendation?

Believe it or not, not everyone you ask to write an LOR for you will write a positive one. I have personally witnessed this firsthand while serving on the admissions committee at Yale. Why does this happen? In my experience, many applicants look at the requirement of obtaining three LORs simply as an annoying box to be checked off on the application instead of putting thought into who would provide you with the best (favorable) recommendation. Unfortunately, some of you will also wait until the last minute and feel pressured to ask *anyone* to write your LOR to meet the requirement.

Let me provide you with some tips on how to obtain the best LOR:

1. You must know how to ask for it. I recommend you ask the potential referrer: "Professor Jones, do you feel you can write a *strong and favorable* letter of recommendation for my candidacy to PA school?" By asking this way, Professor Jones may feel a particular obligation to commit to writing a *solid and favorable* letter.

   If Professor Jones feels that he cannot commit to writing a strong and favorable LOR supporting your candidacy, he will likely refuse. However, his refusal may be a blessing in disguise, as you won't be surprised to find out that Professor Jones wrote an *unfavorable* letter. In addition, his refusal will provide you with an opportunity to find another referee who *will* provide a positive LOR.

2. You should know this person well and feel confident that she knows you well enough to make specific comments on your qualities to become a competent PA student.

3. You must ask the referrer early in the application process to write the recommendation letter. Be comfortable enough with each person you choose so you can politely nudge them if the deadline is approaching and the letter is not submitted.

4. Make it easy for the referrer to write the letter. For example, provide bullet points on your qualities that the referrer can place directly into the letter. See Appendix 5 for a list of effective phrases and the five categories that make an LOR effective.

5. Write it yourself! That's right, if you want a solid and positive LOR, who is better to write it than you? You may think this is a bit forward, but it's a common practice. Of course, you must first *feel out* the person you ask to write your LOR. Get a sense of how they might react to your request. You may want to say, "Sue, I know you are extremely busy, and your time is valuable. I would certainly be willing to compose a draft letter, and you could make any changes you feel appropriate." Now, if you know Sue well, you should be comfortable with this proposal.

   In my experience, I always feel grateful when someone volunteers to write his own LOR. Why? I have a hectic schedule, and if I like this person, I want to do a great job with my recommendation; it will take some time to create the letter. I welcome any help. Of course, if I disagree with anything in the letter, I will make the appropriate changes.

In the next chapter, we will cover one of the CASPA application's most stressful components: the essay.

[CHAPTER 6]

The Essay: Your Ticket to the Interview

Your physician assistant (PA) school essay may be the most critical piece of medical writing that you will ever accomplish. I have been reviewing PA school application essays for over 25 years, both as an admissions committee (ADCOM) member and a PA school applicant coach. On many occasions, the only thing standing between you and an invitation to interview is your essay.

In this chapter, I adapt most of the information from *IvyEssays* (IvyEssays.com.) *IvyEssays* are admissions experts who've spent years integrating the advice of admissions counselors from the nation's top schools. They have also compiled thousands of essays from successful applicants.

I partnered with *IvyEssays* several years ago, and we've helped hundreds of PA school applicants. We get applicant's interviews!

PA school applicants can utilize the services of *IvyEssays* by going directly to IvyEssays.com. When you submit your essay for editing, be sure to mention my name in the comments box, so *IvyEssays* will know exactly how to edit your PA school essay.

GENERAL TIPS FOR WRITING SUCCESSFUL ESSAYS

During the first, quick look at your file (transcripts, science and non-science Grade Point Averages [GPAs], Medical College Admission Test Graduate

Record Examination [GRE] scores, application, recommendations, and personal statement), what the ADCOM seeks is essentially the same:

- Proven ability to succeed
- Evident intellectual ability, analytical, and critical thinking skills
- Evidence that this person can make not just an excellent PA student but a competent PA.

But what they look for when they hone in on your essay is much more than this. Therefore, I will discuss the things typically unanimously listed as the most important by ADCOMs.

Express Motivation

Your application to PA school is a testimony to your desire to become a PA ultimately. The ADCOM will look to your essay to see that you've demonstrated the obvious—but not so simple—the question, *why?* Therefore, you must be able to explain your motivation for attending PA school.

"I look for a sustained understanding of why the candidate wants to enter medicine, how they've tested their interest, and how they've prepared for PA school."

"Touch on your passion for pursuing medicine. For many of you, medicine is akin to a calling, and it is compelling for the evaluator to sense that they are hearing and responding to the same motivation."

I will offer much advice in the upcoming pages and pepper you with plenty of "dos" and "don'ts." But, in the midst of all of this, whatever you do, don't lose sight of the ultimate goal of the essay: you must convince the ADCOM that you belong at their PA school. Use everything I tell you as a means to this end, so step back from the details regularly to remind yourself of the big picture:

"The essay is the venue for the candidate to make the argument as to why they, among all the qualified candidates, should be admitted to PA school and the eventual practice of medicine."

Demonstrate Effective Communication Skills

Another obvious function of the essay is to showcase your language abilities and writing skills.

"In the essay, I want you to have a clear sense that you understand and communicate why you are a compelling candidate."

"Especially if you did some or all of their prerequisite coursework in another country, the ADCOM would look to the essay to ensure strong English language skills."

At this level, good writing skills are expected, not sought. So while a beautifully written essay isn't going to get you into PA school, a poorly written one could keep you out of it.

Beyond showcasing your writing abilities and demonstrating your motivation, what else can the essay do for you? Let's take a look at what else the committee hopes to find when they pick your essay.

Discuss Your Soft Skills

Let the rest of your application—not the personal statement—speak for your *hard* skills and achievements [i.e., your academic excellence, your great MCAT (GRE) scores, your class rank]. They seek in the essay some specific *soft* skills such as maturity, empathy, compassion, depth, and motivation. These qualities were rated exceptionally high in the medical community—more so than any other graduate-level program we studied (Table 6.1).

These qualities are not quantifiable, and therefore not easily demonstrated.

All of the essays I have in my database demonstrate in one way or another that the writers have the *soft* skills necessary to be good medical providers. A few of them even come right out and say it:

"Motivation, independence, maturity, precisely those qualities my experiences in Eastern Europe instilled, will be essential to a fruitful career."

Table 6.1. Qualities Rated High in the Medical Field

1	2	3
Motivation	Diversity	Sensitivity
Commitment	Uniqueness	Communication skills
Sincerity	Interest	Humanitarian beliefs
Honesty	Compassion	Enthusiasm
Maturity	Empathy	Creativity

But when mentioned directly, the applicant must be careful to support the claims with clear evidence from their personal experience. Unfortunately, they often just let their achievements speak for themselves, and the qualities they demonstrate are inferred.

Be Real

I didn't list the items by order of importance—if they were, I would list this category first. More than any specific skill or characteristic, the ADCOM seeks more than anything else in the personal statement is a real, live human being:

"The members of a medical admissions committee are responsible for choosing the next generation of physician assistants. These are the people who will heal our children, cure our parents, and save lives. So, please put it in that perspective, and the responsibility they feel is enormous. For this reason, they're going to choose to accept someone they think they know, trust, and like."

In light of this, it might not surprise you that when I asked ADCOMs and PA students for their #1 piece of advice regarding the essay, we received the same response almost every time. Although expressed in many different ways (be honest, sincere, unique, personal, etc.), it all came down to the same point: *Be Yourself!*

My #1 piece of advice is: BE YOURSELF WHEN YOU WRITE THE ESSAY ... THE MEDICAL PROFESSION IS A LIFETIME COMMITMENT ... LET THEM TRULY KNOW WHAT DRIVES YOU TOWARD IT!

Unfortunately, achieving this level of communication in writing does not come naturally to everyone. But that does not mean you can't learn to do it. Once you understand the essential factors that go into personable writing, you will see that it is not as hard as it seems.

NOTE: Part of what can make this kind of writing seem so tricky is that it is tough to gauge the image you are projecting through your writing. Even if you have followed every tip in this chapter, it is a good idea to have someone objective—preferably someone who doesn't already know you well—read it over when you have finished. Ask them if they got a sense of the kind of person you are or if they could picture you as they were reading. How accurate is their description to the one you're trying to present? Then ask them if they feel comfortable if the person they pictured would care for them in a life or death situation.

Be Personal

The only way to let the ADCOM see you as an individual is to make your essay personal. When you do this, your essay will automatically be more exciting and engaging, helping it stand out from the hundreds of others the committee will be reviewing that week.

After reading hundreds of essays since 1996, I would tell people a couple of crucial things. First, make it personal. The most boring, dry essays are those that go on about how they love science and working with people and want to serve humanity, but give few personal details that provide a sense of what the applicant is like.

Personalize your essay as much as possible—generic essays are not only boring to read, they're also a waste of time because they don't tell you anything about the applicant that helps you get to know them better.

But what does it mean to make your essay personal? It means that you drop the formalities and write about something significant to you. It means that you include a story or anecdote taken from your life, using lots of details and colorful imagery to give it life. And it means, above all, being completely honest.

The following example excerpt is an example. The writer begins by recollecting her experience with anorexia and her admiration for the doctor who saved her life. But it is more than this story that makes her essay real; it is how she describes her experiences. She uses a natural, personal tone throughout the essay, for example, when she describes herself while volunteering at an AIDS clinic.

"I am constantly reminded about how much I have to learn. I look at a baby and notice its cute pudgy toes. Dr. V. plays with it while conversing with its mother, and in less than a minute, has noted its responsiveness, strength, and attachment to its parent and checked its reflexes, color, and hydration. Gingerly I search for the tympanic membrane in the ears of a cooperative child and touch an infant's warm, soft belly, willing my hands to have a measure of Dr. V.'s competence."

It is her admittance that she doesn't know everything she needs to know, coupled with the picture she paints of herself noticing a baby's *cute pudgy toes* and *gingerly* searching in *the ear of a cooperative child* and touching *an infant's warm, soft belly*. It is hard not to feel the individual behind the one who painted such a vivid portrayal using personal details.

Just as this writer did not rely on her tale of anorexia to make her essay personal, as one admissions officer put it:

"A personal epiphany, tragedy, life change, or earth-shattering event is not essential to a strong essay."

I can't stress this point enough. Personal does not have to mean heavy, or emotional, or even inspiring. It is a small minority of students who will genuinely have had a life-changing event to mention. Perhaps they had spent time living abroad or have experienced death or disease from proximity. But this is the exception, not the rule.

Students who rely too heavily on these weighty experiences often do themselves an injustice. They usually don't think about what has touched them or interests them because they are preoccupied with the topic they believe will impress the committee. For example, they write about their grandfather's death because they think that only death (or the emotional equivalent) is significant enough to make them seem deep and mature. But what often happens is they rely on the experience itself to speak for them and never explain what it meant to them or give a solid example of how it changed them. In other words, they don't make it personal.

Use Details

To make your essay personal, learn from the example above and use details. Your goal is to *show, not tell,* who you are by backing your claims with real past experiences.

Essays only help if they are unique and enable the interviewer to get a sense of you as a person, based on examples and scenarios, and ideas, rather than lists of what you may have done. The readers want to know who this person is, not what they've done, although the two are interrelated.

The keywords from the quote are *examples, scenarios,* and *ideas.* Using details means getting specific. Every point that you make needs to be backed up by particular instances taken from your experience. It is these details that make your story memorable, unique, and engaging.

Look at the detail used in the following example. The writer takes care to describe herself gently rocking her first patient, *taking care not to disturb the jumbled array of tubes that overwhelmed his tiny body.* She has *worked with everything from papier mache to popsicle sticks.* In her ward, the children talk about *Nintendo or the latest Disney movie.* The children are the difference between a personal, stimulating treatment of a story and a yawn-inducing account attributed to many applicants.

Tell a Story

Telling a story always makes for more exciting reading, and it usually conveys something more personal than blanket statements like *I want to help people.*

Incorporating a story into your essay can be a great way to make it fascinating and enjoyable. The safest and most common method of integrating a story into an essay is to tell the story first, then step back into the role of narrator and explain why you included the story and the lessons you learned. This method works because it forces you to begin with the action, which is a surefire way to get the reader's attention and keep them reading.

Many of the essay examples in Appendix 6 make effective use of storytelling. One begins with a storm at sea, one with a tale of stage fright before a theater performance, and one with a newspaper clipping about the writer as a child. Another writer takes an even more creative approach to the story method by incorporating the story of a prehistoric woman whose bones he has analyzed throughout the entire essay. All these writers understood that a story is an excellent way to grab the reader's attention. It should always relate to the motivation to attend PA school or the ability to succeed once admitted.

Be Honest

This last tip comes with no caveats. Uphold it without exception. Nothing could be simpler, more straightforward, or more crucial than this: be honest, forthright, and sincere.

Admissions officers have zero tolerance for hype. If you try to be something that you're not, it will be transparent to the committee. You will come off as immature at best and as unethical at worst. For example, if you say that one of your favorite hobbies is playing chess, you better have a favorite opening move; your interviewer may be an expert player and may want to swap techniques!

I served on Yale's ADCOM and can say that it is so important, to be honest. The students will often be asked about the personal statement when interviewing, and it's painfully apparent when they exaggerate or are overly dramatic when recounting their experiences.

When you are honest about your motivation and goals, you will be more personable and genuine. One essayist, for example, begins:

"When I entered Dartmouth College in 1987, I was amazed by the large number of students already labeled as "pre-meds." I wondered how those students were able to decide with such certainty that they wanted to study medicine. I imagined that they all must have known from a very early age that they would one day be great clinicians. Unfortunately, I had no such clues, and if asked what I wanted to be when I grew up, I would have said that I wanted to be an Olympic skier or soccer player."

Because of the plethora of essays that begin: "I've wanted to be a PA for as long as I can remember ..." this writer's honesty must have been refreshing and memorable.

SELECTING AN ESSAY TOPIC

Getting Started

To get the most benefit out of this section, put your anxieties aside. Don't think about what the ADCOM wants, don't worry about grammar or style, and don't worry about what anyone thinks. Worries like these hamper spontaneity and creativity. Focus instead on writing quickly and recording every thought you have the instant you have it. You will know that you are performing these exercises correctly if you are relaxing and having fun.

Stream of Consciousness

Take 20 minutes to answer each of the questions: Who are you? What do you want? Start with whatever comes to mind first, and without pausing for the entire time. Don't limit yourself to any one area of your life, such as your career. Just let yourself go, be honest, and have fun. You might be surprised by what kind of results can come from this type of free association.

Morning Pages

If you have the discipline to practice this technique for a week, you may end up doing it for the rest of your life. Keep a paper and a pen at your bedside. Set your alarm clock 20 minutes early, and when you are still in bed and groggy with sleep, start writing. Write about anything that comes to mind as fast as you can, and do not stop until you have filled a page or two.

Journal Writing

Keep a journal for a few weeks, especially if you are stuck and your brainstorming seems to be going nowhere. Record not what you do each day but your responses and thoughts about each day's experiences.

Top Tens

Write down your top 10 favorites in the following areas: movies, books, songs, musicians, sports, paintings, historical places, and famous people. Then, step back and look at the lists objectively:

- What do they say about you?
- Which favorites are you most passionate about?
- How have these favorites affected your outlook, opinions, or direction?

Free-Flow Writing

Choose a word from your questions such as *influence, strengths, career, diversity,* or *goals,* and brainstorm around it. Set a timer for 10 minutes and write without stopping. Write down everything you can think of that relates to the topic, including any single word that comes to mind.

Assessing Yourself

Hopefully, the exercises in the last section successfully stirred your thoughts and animated your pen. If so, then it is time to impose more focus on your brainstorming. The following exercises help you do just that. They concentrate on finding the specific points and details, allowing you to better formulate answers to your questions. But as you work on them, be sure to retain the open mind and creative attitude you approached in the last exercises.

First, make a list of all the questions you have to answer for each school, leaving plenty of space next to each. Then, work on the following exercises proactively, keeping these questions in mind as you write. When you uncover a point or example that you want to use in response to one of them, note it next to the question, and then return to the brainstorming. If you can apply one situation or experience to multiple questions, do so. Don't censor yourself. More is better at this stage of the writing process—you can worry about honing and culling later. The objective now is to accumulate multiple items for each question.

The Chronological Method

Start from childhood and record any significant or pivotal experiences that you remember. Go from grade to grade, and job to job, noting any critical lessons learned, achievements reached, painful moments endured, or obstacles overcome. Also, include your feelings about those occurrences as you remember them. If you are a visual person, it might help to draw a timeline. Do not leave out any significant event.

Because so many questions ask about your past, this exercise will help you uncover material you can use in several places. A few schools will ask you directly about your childhood and highlight a youth's memory. Don't automatically discount memories that you think will seem trite or silly. A childhood memory could be used, for example, to demonstrate a long-standing passion or to emphasize how an aspect of your character is so ingrained that it has been with you since youth.

Assess Your Accomplishments

Write down anything you are proud of doing, no matter how small or insignificant it might seem. Do not limit your achievements to your career. If you have overcome a difficult personal obstacle, be sure to list this too. If something is important to you, it speaks volumes about who you are and what makes you tick. Some accomplishments will be obvious, such as an achievement that received public acknowledgment. Others are less so, and often the defining moments of our lives are those we are inclined to dismiss.

List Your Skills

Do a similar assessment of the skills that you did for your accomplishments. Begin by looking at the actions you listed for the last exercise and documenting the skills that these accomplishments demonstrate. When you have a list of words, start brainstorming on specific scenarios that demonstrate these skills. Pretend that you are defending these skills in front of a panel of judges. Stop when you have proven each point to the best of your ability. Some of your skills will be obvious, such as artistic, musical, or athletic abilities. Others will be more subtle (but just as important!).

Analyze Personality Traits

Take advantage of the often fuzzy distinction between skills and personality traits. If you have trouble listing and defending your skills, shift the focus to your qualities and characteristics instead.

Make a few columns on a sheet of paper. In the first one, list some adjectives you would use to describe yourself. In the next one, list the words your best friend would use. Then, use the other columns for other types of people—perhaps one for your favorite teacher and another for family members or classmates.

When you finish, see which words come up the most often. Then group them and list the different situations in which you have exhibited these characteristics. How effectively can you illustrate or prove that you possess these qualities? Again, establishing your points is essential.

Note Major Influences

You can refer back to your *Top Ten* lists for help getting started with this exercise. Did a particular book or quote make you rethink your life? Was there a specific person who shaped your values and views? Relationships can be good material for an essay, particularly one that challenges you to look at people differently. Perhaps you had a wise and generous mentor from whom you learned a great deal. Have you had an experience that changed how you see the world or defines who you are? What details of your life, notable achievements, and pivotal events have helped shape you and influenced your goals?

Identify Your Goals

The first step of this exercise is to let loose and write down anything that comes to mind in response to the following questions: What are your wildest dreams? What did you want to be when you were a kid? What would it be if you could do or be anything right now, regardless of skill, money, or other restrictions? Think as broadly as you wish, and do not limit yourself to career goals. Will you have kids? What kind of house will you live in, and what types of friends will you have? What would you do if you were so rich that you didn't have to work?

Identifying Your Themes

Part of what makes the personal statement so tricky is that you need to do so much in one essay. Unlike the college application essay, where your motivation is unquestioned, your goals can remain undefined. Unlike other graduate programs where you must write multiple essays in response to specific questions, writing a personal statement requires incorporating numerous themes in one composition. Combining the pieces can be tricky.

You need to incorporate three primary themes. The first addresses the question, "Why do you want to be a PA?" The second address "Why are you unique, different, or exceptional?" And the third, "Why are you qualified?" and "What experience have you had?"

There are several different ways to approach each one of these themes. The more common of these approaches are outlined below, with tips and advice on handling each one.

Theme 1: Why I Want to be a PA?

Many people look back to cite the moment of their initial inspiration. However, some people have wanted to be a PA for so long they don't even know what originally inspired them. To incorporate this theme, look back to the material you gathered in the last section, specifically in response to *The Chronological Method, Note Major Influences, and Identify Your Goals.* Then, ask yourself these questions:

1. How old was I when I first wanted to be a PA? Was there a defining moment? Was there ever any ambivalence?
2. Did a specific person inspire me?
3. What kind of PA do I want to be, and how does that tie into my motivation?

Here are a few of the common ways that students incorporate this theme: "I've always wanted to be a PA."

AKA: "I've wanted to be a PA since I was ...," and "Everyone has always said I'd be a good PA."

I've always wanted to be a PA is perhaps the most common approach of all. The secret to doing it well is to show, not just tell, why you want to be a PA. You can't just say it and expect it to stand on its own.

Additionally, the *I've always wanted to be a PA* essay has been done to death. Therefore, I think such candidates need to be careful that their decision was not only a preadolescent one but also has been tested over the years and approached maturely.

Supply believable details from your life to make your desire real to the reader. One secret to avoiding the *here we go again* reaction is to be particularly careful with your first line. Starting with "I've wanted to be a PA since ..." makes them cringe. It's an easy line to fall back on, but admissions officers have read this sentence more times than they care to count—don't add to the statistic.

"My Dad is a PA . . ."

This approach to the "Why I want to be a PA" theme is dangerous for a different reason.

It's a prejudice of mine, but the legacy essay, the one that reads, "My Dad and my Mom are PAs, and I should be too," makes me suspect immaturity. I envision a young person who can't think for themselves or make up their minds.

However, not every ADCOM member has this opinion. The point isn't to avoid admitting that your parent is a PA; it is to avoid depending on that as the sole reason you want to go to PA school. If a parent indeed was your inspiration, then explain why he inspired you. One essay in our database takes a unique approach—he tells of how he initially revolted about becoming a PA because of family pressure. His story about how he eventually came around makes for an exciting and convincing read.

"My PA Changed My Life!"

AKA: "Being a patient made me want to become a PA."

Some people are motivated to become PAs because they have had a personal experience of illness or disability.

I had a student who grew up with a chronic illness. She spent much time with physicians and PAs throughout her young life. In her personal statement, she wrote about this continuing experience and how the medical professionals treated her. She wrote of her admiration of them as well as her understanding that they couldn't yet cure her. Her essay jumped off the page as being unique to her. The essay provided a compelling testament of her desire to join the people who had been so crucial to her life.

If your personal experience with the medical industry sincerely motivates you to attend PA school, then do write about it. The problem is that many students fall back on this topic even when it doesn't hold particularly true for them. I can't stress enough that you do not have to have a life-defining ability or a dramatic experience to have an exciting statement. ADCOMs receive piles of accident- and illness-related essays, and the ones that seem insincere stick out like sore thumbs (pun intended!) and do not reflect well on you as a candidate.

"My orthodontist changed my life!" "My dentist gave my smile back!" These themes are indeed valid but go beyond what particular aspect of the profession intrigues you. Do you understand how many years of study your orthodontist had to endure to reach his level of practice? Have you observed your dentist for any significant amount of time? Do you know that the profession now is much different than it was when he was starting? Have you given any thought to the danger of infectious diseases to all health care professionals? Present a well-organized, complete essay.

One of the essayists in our database begins with a line that is often overused and makes it the subject of the first paragraph. What makes it work is that he moves briskly in the next section to demonstrate that he balanced his initial inspiration with real hospital experience. The experience taught him that being a PA is more about hard work and commitment than about the good feeling of being cured or curing.

Another of our essayists describes her experience with illness in vivid language to capture the reader's interest:

"The morning of New Year's Day, 1978, was bright and sunny. Refreshed from a good night's sleep, I lifted the blankets, rose to my feet, and collapsed, unable to walk."

She does not dwell on the experience, though, and like the others, provides plenty of further evidence of her sincere motivation.

Another demonstrates the most personal patient experience of them all: she suffered from anorexia. She "slowly came to realize that my pediatrician had saved my life—despite my valiant efforts to the contrary." Her story works because she tells her story objectively and with no intention to manipulate the reader's emotions.

"My Mom Had Cancer"

This theme is just a variation of "I was a patient myself," and the same advice applies: If a loved one's battle with illness, trauma, or a disability is what inspired your wish to become a PA, then, by all means, mention it. But don't dwell on it, don't over-dramatize, and don't let it stand as your sole motivation—show that you've done your research and you understand the life of a PA and choose it for a variety of reasons.

Two of our essayists briefly mention their sister's struggles (one with cancer and one mentally challenged), but neither spends more than a couple of sentences on the subject. Another begins with the story of a teacher who has AIDS. What validates this focus is the writer's subsequent involvement as a volunteer at an HIV clinic—without this evidence to prove her sincerity, the poignancy of the situation is doubtful, and the essay considerably weakened.

"I Want to Help People"

It is common and natural to cite a desire to help people. Many of the essayists in our database do just this. Perhaps the most poignant and convincing of the group is the applicant who writes of his involvement with three boys as part of a volunteer program. It is easy to see how a person would make a kind, caring, and involved PA. Another essayist compares being a PA to being a minister—it rings sincere when we discover that he is an elder in his church.

The Medical Dichotomy

One of the major draws of the medical field is the dualistic nature of combining hard-core science with the softer side of helping people. People describe this in many ways: some describe it as a dichotomy of science to art. To others, it's intellectualism to humanism, theory to application, research to creativity, or qualitative to social skills. No matter how you choose to phrase it, if you mention the dichotomy, then be sure to touch on your qualifications and experience in both areas.

Theme 2: Why Am I an Exceptional Person?

This theme is often tied in closely with *why I am a qualified person?* Be very clear on the difference, though the latter focuses specifically on your experience (medical or otherwise) that qualifies you to be a better PA student. In contrast, this one focuses strictly on you as a person. Committees are always on the lookout for well-rounded candidates. They want to see that you are interesting, involved, and tied to the community around you.

To help you think about supporting this theme, look at the answers to the exercises from the last chapter and ask yourself: *What makes me different? Do I have any unique talents or abilities that might make me more attractive? How will my skills and personality traits add diversity to the class? What makes me stand out from the crowd? How will this help me to be a better PA and student?*

If you are creative, you'll be able to take whatever makes you different—even a flaw—and turn it to your advantage.

One student wrote about her experience as a childhood *klutz* and how many accidents kept her continually in medical care. The care she received was the impetus to her desire to be a PA and made her essay entertaining, sincere, and eminently credible.

Note that the candidate in this example tied her experience into her desire to become a PA. Be sure to do this with practically every point you make in your essay.

The Talented Among Us

If you are one of a lucky few with outstanding talent or ability, now is no time to hide it. Whether you are a star athlete, an opera singer, or a violin virtuoso, by all means, make it a focus of your essay.

These people can be some of the strongest candidates. Assuming, always, that they've excelled in the required preparatory coursework, the other strengths can take them over the top. Athletes, musicians, etc., can make the compelling case of excellence, achievement, discipline, mastering a subject/talent, and leveraging their abilities. PA programs are full of these types—they thrive by bringing high achievers who possess intellectual knowledge into their realm.

If you plan to focus on a strength outside the field of medicine, your challenge is to tie the experience into your motivation for becoming a PA.

One of our essayists describes an African drumming performance during a Catholic mass and then ties back to the musical theme nicely in the last line. Music was a profound interest in another writer's life, and she rightly devotes her theme to the healing power of music and her study of musical therapy.

Another essayist draws a compelling portrait of an avid skier and swimmer and effectively ties her interest in sports to medicine through her experience as a lifeguard and a member of the emergency medical ski team.

Students of Diversity

If you are diverse in any sense of the word: if you are an older applicant, a minority, a foreign applicant, or disabled, use it to your advantage by showing what your unique background will bring to the school and the practice of medicine. Some admissions officers, however, warn against using minority status as a qualification instead of quality. If you fall into this trap, your diversity will work against you.

You are building a bridge between the two. If you are a *student of diversity*, then, of course, use it. But don't harp on it for its own sake or think that being diverse by itself is enough to get you in—that will only make the reader feel manipulated, and it will show that you didn't know how to take advantage of a good opportunity.

So be sure you tie it in with your motivation or argument for why it makes you a better candidate; you will be standing on safe ground.

Late Comers and Career Switchers

Luckily for all of us, you needn't be a minority, a foreign applicant, disabled, athlete, or musician to be considered diverse. There are, for example, those who have had experience in or prepared themselves for totally different fields. One management consultant wrote about his desire to switch careers. Another begins by telling how miserable he was as a branch manager for a marketing corporation. Another woman writes about how she always planned to go into public health, and yet another originally wanted to be a veterinarian. Yet, they all give brief reasons to shift into medicine and show evidence of sincere and intensive preparation for their new chosen field.

English Majors and Theater People

Not everyone accepted to PA school has a hard-core science background. One essayist initially wanted to be a writer and comments persuasively on the similarities between analyzing literature and medical research. He takes this one step further when discussing the creative versus the analytical approach to medicine and his lofty ambition of building a bridge between the two. One essay opens with the author's involvement in a play and openly admits that science and math initially turned her off. Another was a Classics major, and another reveals that she *turned away from science during my undergraduate years.*

The secret of all these essays is that they know how to turn their potential weaknesses into strengths. For example, they point out that communication is an integral part of being a PA and discuss the advantages of their well-rounded backgrounds. However, they are also cautious about demonstrating their motivation and qualifications in detail. Nevertheless, the writers provide solid evidence to offset worries that a non-science background doesn't necessarily equate to an unrealistic view of a PA's life. They show their ability to cope with science courses will not be compromised.

Can I Be too Well-Rounded?

Some people have talents, abilities, or experience in so many areas that they risk coming across as unfocused or undedicated. When handled deftly, though, you bring your many sides together, and what could have hurt you ends up setting you apart instead. One of our essayists does a terrific job of this. She was an Art History major, active in varsity sports, health education, and traveling. In addition, she'd been an au pair in Iceland and an exchange student and intern in France. Yet, she manages to present all of this in a short, pointed essay. She uses the concept of *connections* as her theme. She relates systems of connections to the human body and her diverse activities, emphasizing how they all come together to form a coherent and unique whole.

Taking Advantage of International Experience

Many applicants have international experience. So, while it may not set you apart in a unique way, it is always worthwhile to demonstrate your cross-cultural understanding and sensitivity. Many in our database have written descriptions of their foreign experience ranging from volunteering in Africa, Brazil, and Honduras to au pairing in Iceland to opera singing in Paris. One essay is influential in the area of international experience. This exceptional man worked as a farmhand in Hungary and an orderly in the Former Soviet Union, financed by the first hospital in Estonia and organized a mission to deliver medical supplies to refugees in Bosnia.

Notice again, though, that all these essayists went beyond simply writing about their experiences. They related these experiences either to their motivation or qualifications. Don't expect the committee to make these leaps for you—you need to put it in your own words and make the connection clear.

Religion

Some admissions counselors advise avoiding mention of religion altogether. Others say faith gives the applicant an advantage by setting them apart and stressing values and commitment. Faith is a somewhat touchy subject area, best left to the individual choice. A few of our essayists mention religion to varying degrees. One was a missionary for the Church of Latter-day Saints for 2 years, and another was an elder of the same. The last merely mentions Bible study in passing, so to speak, it still sheds light on what is probably an essential part of her life.

Theme 3: Why Am I a Qualified Person?

The last central theme deals with your experience and qualifications for attending PA school and becoming a good provider. Having direct hospital, allied health experience, or research experience is always the best evidence you can give. If you haven't, then consider what other experience you have that is related. Perhaps you've been a volunteer or tutored English as a second language? Were you a teaching assistant? The rule to follow here is: if you have done it, use it.

Hospital/Clinical Experience

Direct experience with patients is probably the best kind to have in your essay. What is essential to notice in the essays in my database is that applicants cite any type or amount of experience, no matter how insignificant it might appear. Some essayists even cite experience they gained in high school. Many are volunteers, some as HIV counselors, some in emergency rooms, some as lab assistants, and some simply escorted patients to their correct rooms.

Research Experience

A word of caution: don't focus solely on your research topic—your essay will become impersonal at best and downright dull at worst. Watch out for overuse of what non-science types refer to as *medical garble*. If it's necessary for the description of your project, then, of course, you have no choice. But throwing medical terms around just because you can won't impress anyone. Good writers can delve into the use of scientific and medical terms, but they also spend plenty of time away from them as well, sounding like real human beings.

Unusual Medical Experience

Even if you haven't put in X number of hours a week at a clinic or spent a term on a research project, you might still have the medical experience that counts. Perhaps you cared for your sick grandmother or the day you saved the man at the adjacent table from choking in a restaurant. It doesn't even matter if you were unsuccessful (maybe, despite your valiant efforts, the man at the table didn't survive); if it was meaningful to you, then it was relevant. But, on the other hand, one relays a fascinating success story: the writer became a medical provider by default to a village in Honduras for summer, even though she had no formal training, no experience, and her only supply was *a $15 Johnson & Johnson medical kit.*

Nonmedical Experience

Your experience doesn't even have to be medically related to be relevant. Many successful applicants cite nonmedical volunteer experience as evidence of their willingness to help and heal the human race. Almost every one of our essayists was either a volunteer or a tutor at some point in their lives.

Developing a Strategy

Once you have decided how to incorporate the various themes into your essay, the last step is to develop a strategy—or in other words, figure out how you are going to weave your themes together into a coherent whole. Here's some advice you don't often get: don't think about this one too much. What's nice about strategy is that it tends to fall into place by itself once you develop an outline and start writing, which is what the next section is all about. So what I offer here is no more than a couple of tips for you to consider—but not to worry too much about it. In the end, there is no more I can tell you about strategy without knowing more about your personality.

Strategy Tip 1: Keep the School in Mind

Most students write generic personal statements. These essays get sent to every school that you choose on your CASPA application. That's fine, and to a degree, unavoidable. But it always impresses me when you do your research and shows in your essays why you are a good fit for that particular school (especially on supplemental applications for PA school).

Know the schools to which you are applying and know what they look for in an applicant. Some schools are heavily diversity-based, some only want in-state residents, some like the heaviest science preparation possible. Do your homework!

Don't be lazy about this! At the very least, you can find out about the school's general reputation by scanning the website (also Google, Facebook, and YouTube). Better, though, is to research the faculty and familiarize yourself with a school's specific strengths. The information you gather becomes fodder for the statement and will be crucial later when you interview.

Strategy Tip 2: Keep the Rest of Your Application in Mind

Step back and take a look at your entire application package. Imagine that you are the admissions officer looking at it for the first time. What do the test scores, the science and non-science GPA, the kind of courses you took, the recommendations, the extracurriculars, and the supplemental materials say about you? Do you feel it presents a complete picture of you? If it doesn't, what can you include in your essay to round it out? Also, note if there are any obvious red flags.

I look to the personal statement to explain gaps or discrepancies in your background. If you don't provide that information, you leave room for the committee to speculate. Anything the candidate offers is bound to be better than the committee hypothesizes in its absence.

Also, note redundancies. Don't recapitulate in your essay that which can be found elsewhere in the application. Don't repeat your GPA or your GRE score, no matter how impressive. And, as noted previously, don't try to cram in a prose listing of your activities and accomplishments when there is space elsewhere. It isn't exciting and shows that you don't know how to take advantage of an excellent opportunity to showcase your personal qualities.

Strategy Tip 3: Avoid Discussing Medical Issues

Though known to come up during interviews, a discussion of medical issues is not often attempted in the essay and not generally advised. There are many reasons for this: (1) the essay is supposed to be about you, not about issues, (2) your audience likely knows more about the issues than you do, (3) with only 5,000 characters to do the issue justice, you will probably end up biting off more than you can chew, and (4) you risk offending someone on the committee. Of course, the natural exception to this rule is if a medical issue featured prominently in your decision to become a PA. One essayist, for example, cites the public health care debate as one of her primary draws to the field.

Discussing your negative views of the medical field in your statement is dangerous. But, like anything, some do it well. One of my essayists, for example, discusses what he perceives as a conflict in the medical world and demonstrates how he will contribute to its resolution. Though he deals with what he sees as a negative conflict in the medical arena, he discusses it objectively and tactfully.

Another essayist doesn't give her opinion on medical issues. Still, she does cite the bad experience she had with her pediatrician as a child as her chief motivation for her to do a better job as a medical provider herself. Both of these examples discuss their potential roles in the resolution of the conflict. Even when you keep these tactics in mind, though, the best advice here is definitely, *when in doubt, to leave it out.*

An Alternative Approach

No matter how hard and fast these rules regarding theme and strategy may seem, there will always be applicants who will decide to toss it all to the wind and take a completely different approach. The writer of one essay, for example, incorporates none of the mentioned themes into his personal statement. He doesn't talk about his motivation or qualifications for attending PA school. He only says PA school once, and even then, it is a single reference made only as an aside. He chose, instead, to focus his entire essay on his experience as a rower at Cambridge University in England.

This is a risky approach and one that students best take with already solid backgrounds. This applicant felt confident that the rest of his application spoke well enough of his qualifications that he could focus entirely on another aspect of his life. And this approach does have the merit of painting a vivid picture of the applicant in his natural surroundings. It gives the reader a strong sense of his character and drive. However, ultimately it is a personal decision. Again, the best way to gauge whether or not the risk is worth taking is by finding a candidate capable of giving you objective and informed Feedback.

Avoiding Pitfalls

Pitfall #1: The Hard-Luck Tale

Some genuinely outstanding essays are about solid emotional experiences such as a childhood struggle with disease or the death of a loved one—some written so effectively that they hold up as role models for all essays.

I had a student who was considered a weak candidate because of poor grades and low test scores. She was African American, and although she had pursued all the right avenues (classes, GREs, volunteer experiences) to prepare herself for PA school, she remained undistinguished as a candidate—until, that is, she wrote her essay. The essay revealed her tremendous and sincere drive. She was from a crime-riddled area of New York City, and several of her siblings died violently. She wrote about her experience and desire to practice medicine in the city and improve the neighborhood where she grew up. It was compelling, believable, and genuinely inspiring.

While it's true that these poignant tales can provide robust evidence of motivation for PA school, they are challenging to do well; handle them with extreme care and sensitivity. And, as I've said before, don't rely on the tale itself to carry you through—you always need to show your motivation clearly.

I might sound harsh, but I'm not too fond of the tales of woe, like the ones that begin with the mother's death from cancer. Frankly, I feel manipulated, and I don't think the personal statement is the proper mode of expression for that kind of emotion.

Pitfall #2: Making Lists

There is a danger inherent in cramming as much of your experience as possible into 5,000 characters. The threat is ending up with what amounts to little more than a listing of your accomplishments.

I've found that PA school applicants can tend to make laundry lists. However, they need to take extra care to tie their interests, motivation, and preparation together and turn it into a readable and credible argument that fits them.

It is not a bad idea to include all the experiences you have had somewhere in your essay. But do it in the context of a story or a personal account.

The essay should never be a summary from a curriculum vitae. But, again, it's dry to read, and again, doesn't offer any additional information about the candidate.

Pitfall #3: Excuses, Excuses

Because GPA and test scores are crucial to the application process, applicants who have fallen short in either area use the essay to justify their poor performances. Using the essay, for this reason, is not always ill-advised. If there is a true anomaly in your record, the committee will look to your essay for an explanation. Applicants who do this topic well provide a brief and mature description of the lapse, then they spend the rest of the essay focusing on their strengths in other areas.

Explaining a bad grade or even a lousy semester can be done with finesse. So I would never give staying away from that as blanket advice. But, please, just don't whine while you're doing it.

The problems come when you try to excuse a problem instead of explaining it. Some applicants, for example, try to justify low test scores by claiming that they are not good test-takers. Well, I hate to break it to them, but PA school is about taking tests. They are a large part of the curriculum and are proven predictors of academic success. So why would admitting flat-out to being a lousy tester ever be a good thing? Other students try to push the blame for a bad grade onto someone else.

Using the essay to make excuses for your overall poor record isn't an excellent way to get ahead. We don't need to hear about the professor who *had a problem with you* or how your organic chemistry professor *wasn't from America*. These types of statements speak volumes about a person's character.

The only way to know for sure that you're not falling into this trap is to ask someone objective to review your essay for you. Even better, find someone who doesn't even know you and ask them to describe back to you the impression they received of the writer.

CREATING THE STRUCTURE

Now that you know what you want your personal statement to say, it is time to start writing. First, set a time limit of no more than a couple of days. The longer the time frame, the more difficult it will be to write your first draft. The point is not to let yourself sit around waiting for inspiration to strike. As one admissions officer put it, "Some of the worst writing ever crafted has been done under the guise of inspiration."

Relieve some of the pressure of writing by reminding yourself that this is just a draft. Rid yourself of the notion that your essay can be perfect on the first try. Don't agonize over a particular word choice or the phrasing of an idea—you will have plenty of time to perfect the essay later. For now, the most important thing is to get some words on paper.

Creating an Outline

You are probably familiar by now with the structure of the traditional outline taught in grade school:

Paragraph #1: (Introduction which contains the central idea)
Paragraph #2:

- Topic sentence that ties into the central idea

- First supporting point
- Evidence for point

Paragraph #3:

- Topic sentence which links the above paragraph to the next
- Second supporting point
- Evidence for point

Paragraph #4:

- Topic sentence which links the above paragraph to the next
- Third supporting point
- Evidence for point

Paragraph #5:

(Conclusion which reiterates the central idea and takes it one step further)

Using this outline as a tried and true method is still your best bet. The problem is that it may not allow for the complexities created by the multiple themes you need to incorporate into your essay. Your outline will probably end up looking more complicated than this one, but that is no excuse for not having one. The more complex the essay, the more in need of an outline it will be. Without it, your essay will lack structure. Without structure, your essay will be rambling and ineffective.

Take some time to play with the material you have, put it into different structures, and always offer the best support for your main points. Then, consider the examples below to get ideas for different outlines that you can apply to your statement.

Standard Structure

The standard structure is the most common. I recommend it for use in almost any circumstance. You are applying it as close as you can get at this level to the simple structure outlined above. The general application of the standard format is to introduce the themes and main points in the introduction, use the body of the text to supply one supporting point in each paragraph, and then reiterate your main points in the conclusion in light of the evidence you presented. The following is an example of a pure standard structure used by an applicant who wanted to make the points that she was both interested in and qualified for the medical field on two levels: intellectually and from the standpoint of wanting to help people.

Paragraph #1: (Introduction)

Leading sentence: "Since childhood, my father's inspirational recounts as a cardiologist have captured my heart and interest."

Summary of main points: Introduces *two fundamental tenets* of *working to care and cure,* noting her interest in both the academic and the caring sides of medicine.

Paragraph #2:

Transition sentence: "During my high school and college years, I have explored different areas of community service."

First supporting point: *The writer shows* interest in caring through her community involvement.

Evidence: Tutoring geometry to high-school students and English to recent immigrants.

Paragraph #3:

Transition sentence: "I have also participated in the caring element of the medical profession, providing companionship to patients in the hospital setting."

Second supporting point: Interest in caring, demonstrated by her hospital experience.

Evidence: Volunteer at several hospitals, including the coronary care unit and the cardiac rehabilitation center.

Paragraph #4:

Transition sentence: "It would be simplistic to say that I have chosen to devote my life to the medical profession only because I have a strong desire to help people."

Second supporting point: Also motivated by intellectual exploration.

Evidence: She details her passion for *[making] an intellectual leap and [managing] to land feet first upon a convincing conclusion* and describes the thrill which leaves her *thirsting for the next challenge.*

Paragraph #5:

Transition sentence: "The excitement of intellectual discovery has encouraged me to explore several fields."

Second supporting point: Has a well-rounded academic background.

Evidence: "While my major is biochemistry, my academic interests encompass Asian studies, languages, music, computer science, health care, and environmental policy."

Paragraph #6:

Transition sentence: "My rewarding experiences growing intellectually have not only fueled my passion for exploration and discovery but have also inspired me to share my enthusiasm for learning with others, particularly in the field of science."

Second supporting point: Ties academic interests back to the original theme of caring for people.

Evidence: "To help high-school students embark on their exciting voyages to understand the world around us, I wrote a study guide describing how to approach scientific research and titled it Frontier to emphasize exploration and intellectual discovery."

Paragraph #7:

Transition sentence: "To me, there is only one profession that satisfies both my curiosity and my desire to help those in need."

Reiteration of main points and closing sentence: "Incorporating both the caring, personal, provider-patient relationship and the dynamism of continuous learning, the medical profession is the profession I eagerly embrace, and I believe it is also the best way I can harness my talents and abilities for the benefit of others."

Chronological

Another way to create an outline for your essay is by retelling the events of your life chronologically. The advantage of this approach is that it allows for a more personal approach and helps the committee to know you by turning the focus to you throughout various stages of your life. The drawback is that the points you are trying to make can get lost in the narration of your life.

The following writer uses a chronological structure beginning with the clip of an article describing him as a young boy:

Paragraph #1: (leading Quote)

Leading sentence: "One time, a family cat captured … a moth."

Provides a quote from an article describing him as a boy in 1978.

Paragraph #2: (Introduction)

Transition sentence: "This article, about me as a ten-year-old boy trying to turn a nearby drainage pond into a park, had a misprint—it was a mouse, not a moth."

Explains the quote and makes the main point that he was destined to be a caregiver from a young age.

Paragraph #3:

Transition sentence: "We didn't exactly live on a farm but were in a farming country."

Describes himself and his life as a boy.

Paragraph #4:

Transition sentence: "During this period, we did manage to find time for other things."

Focuses on his multiple activities throughout high-school years.

Paragraph #5:

Transition sentence: "After two semesters at Boise State, I volunteered for two years as a missionary with the Church of Jesus Christ of Latter-Day Saints, going to the California Ventura Mission."

Continues to college-age-years spent as a missionary.

Paragraph #6:

Transition sentence: "Returning to school, my classes included math and sciences (subjects I had shied away from before)—out of curiosity, at first; then, to keep my options open."

Progresses his return to college and his activities and accomplishments from that period.

Paragraph #7:

Transition sentence: "In high school, I had some health problems and seen several doctors."

Steps back to high-school experiences to introduce theme of medicine.

Paragraph #8:

Transition sentence: "This experience soured me in the medical profession."

Interprets experiences described in the last paragraph to explain a late interest in medicine.

Paragraph #9:

Transition sentence: "I pursued psychology and the humanities while growing more fascinated by health, nutrition, and what people I knew had found in 'alternative' approaches to health, including preventive and Eastern medicine."

Talks about his subsequent interest in fields peripheral to medicine.

Paragraph #10:

Transition sentence: "Upon transferring to USC, I found that my view of the medical establishment wasn't accurate—some care more about helping people than about the money or the intellectual pride."

He describes how his interest in medicine solidified while at USC.

Paragraph #11:

Transition sentence: "Throughout my college career, I have had to support myself financially."

He uses the transition to discuss the many jobs he has held throughout the stages in his life.

Incorporating Narrative

Beginning your essay with a story is a common and effective method for catching and keeping the reader's interest. An account is also an excellent way to structure your essay if you want to focus on a single event in your life. In its purest form, a narrative essay does nothing but tell the story. It begins and ends with the action. I do not recommend this for a personal statement. However, at some point, you need to draw the connection from the story to your motivation and qualifications for attending PA school.

The following are some examples of writers who have incorporated narrative into their essays. Notice how each writer provides a clear transition to the rest of their essay.

Essay 1: Paints a picture of herself as a child climbing into her father's dentist chair for treatment. She uses the story to transition into her desire to practice in pediatric dental care.

Essay 2: Begins with a story of working as a deckhand for the Sea Education Association (SEA). Uses story to demonstrate teamwork skills and the importance of community. Transitions with, "Both at sea and on land, I have found great pleasure in the rewards of upholding and enriching the worlds of which I am a part."

Essay 3: Tells the story of her high-school teacher's battle with AIDS. Transitions with: "I entered college, believing that biology could explain to me why life's processes went awry."

Essay 4: Tells the story of unraveling the past of a prehistoric woman by analyzing her bones. Transitions in the last paragraph: "To a large extent, my choice to become a physician assistant is rooted in my desire to continue working *with the human body. But I want to work with the living.*"

Essay 5: Incorporates the story of his attempt to save a life aboard a train in Italy into the middle of his essay rather than at the beginning. He uses it to illustrate the lessons he learned of self-forgetful devotion and the importance of attention to detail.

Notice the variety of circumstances this type of essay can be applied to when comparing these essays. A narrative can span a lifetime or a moment. It does not have to be filled with Hollywood-style action to hold interest. The briefest and most straightforward of events can take on meaning when told effectively. What makes all of these essays effective is their use of detail, description, and direction.

LEADS AND ENDS

Beginnings and endings can be the most challenging part of crafting any piece of writing and, in many ways, the most important. Part of the reason they are so tricky is that writers worry about them too much. There is so much hype on the necessity of thoroughly introducing the subject and ending with sharply drawn conclusions that anxious essayists compensate by going overboard. They feel that, to appear mature and worldly, their essays must contain profound insights and comprehensive observations.

Do not fall into this trap! One of the ADCOM members' biggest complaints was essayists trying to say and do too much in their introductions.

"Just tell the story!" It was repeated like a mantra in response to essayists who were trying too hard to impress. Many of these essays (not included in this chapter) would have been vastly improved had they simply removed their introductions altogether.

Do yourself a favor and forget about beginnings and endings during the first stages of writing. Instead, dive straight into the body of the text without bothering to introduce your themes or set the scene. This technique works because when you have finished writing the rest of your rough draft, you may discover that you don't need an introduction at all. But isn't that risky? Maybe. But believe it or not, forced and unnecessary introductions ruin more essays than the lack of one. Primarily this is because of the misconception of what an introduction is supposed to accomplish.

This is especially true if you are basing your essay around a story. It might feel risky or uncomfortable just letting the story stand on its own without being introduced first, but beginning with action is always a good idea as long as the action is tied closely into the points you are trying to make throughout the rest of the essay.

Leading the Way

The most crucial part of any beginning is, of course, the lead. Leads play the dual role of setting the theme of your essay and engaging the reader. The introduction should not be overly formal or stilted. You do not want an admissions officer to start reading your essay and think, *here we go again.* Although admissions officers will try to give the entire essay a fair reading, they are only human—if you lose them after the first sentence, the rest of your essay will not get the attention it deserves.

Just as you should not worry about your introduction until you have gotten an initial draft on paper, you should not begin writing your lead unless you feel inspired about a particular line. Often, you will find a good one floating around in the middle of your first draft of the essay, so don't waste time worrying about it until you have the bulk of your essay on paper.

There are many different kinds of effective leads. Let's take a look at various tips below.

Standard Lead

Standard leads are the most common leads used. A typical standard lead answers one or more of the six basic questions: who, what, when, where, why, and how. They give the reader an idea of what to expect. A summary lead is a kind of standard lead that answers most of these questions in one sentence. The problem with this kind of lead is that, although it is a logical beginning, it can be dull. The advantage is that it sets your reader up for a focused and well-structured essay. If you live up to that expectation, the impact of your points is heightened. They are also helpful for shorter essays when you need to get to your point quickly.

"Initially, my interest in medicine was due to my family."

"I am interested in participating in a master's level PA program to prepare for a career in medical research."

"My work experiences—ranging from public health projects in rural Latin America to work at Urban battered women's shelters to peer counseling on a college campus—reflect my concern for people's 'health' in a broad sense of the word."

Action Lead

This lead takes the reader into the middle of a piece of the action. Thus, it is perfect for short essays where space needs to be conserved or narrative essays that begin with a story, such as:

"The car swerved to the left."

"She dropped the box on the table and left the room because she didn't want to watch."

"It was opening night. I was about to walk on stage as Ruth in 'The Pirates of Penzance.'"

"As the rusted-out Land Rover made its way cautiously through the dense thicket and cervices in the rocky dirt road, those of us sitting on top were able to peer through the trees at a sublime West African landscape."

"One day in the summer after I graduated from high school, my grandfather took me up to the attic of his house to show me something he thought would be significant for me."

Personal or Revealing Lead

This lead reveals something about the writer. It is always in the first person and usually takes an informal, conversational tone:

"I was not in control of my life, and I was miserable."

"Since my childhood, my father's inspirational recounts as a cardiologist have captured my heart and interest."

"I decided that I wanted to be a health care provider sometime after my four-month incarceration in Columbia Presbyterian Children's Hospital in the winter of 1986-87, as I struggled with anorexia nervosa."

Creative Lead

This lead attempts to add interest by being obtuse or funny. Creative leads can leave you wondering what the essay will be about or make you smile, such as:

"The melody starts slow; a quiet, whirring sound of violins slowly envelopes the hall."

"The beating of an African healing drum resonates throughout all corners of the Catholic church during the weekly five o'clock student mass."

"When I consider my life experiences, I imagine them as interconnected, cooperative, and form-giving systems of bones and joints."

Quotation Lead

This type of lead can be a direct quotation or paraphrase. It is most effective when the quote you choose is unusual, funny, obscure, and not too long. Choose a quote with a meaning you plan to reveal to the reader as the essay progresses. Some admissions officers caution against this kind of lead because it can seem like you are trying to impress them or sound wise. Do not use a proverb or cliché, and do not interpret the quote in your essay. The ADCOM is more interested in how you respond to it and what the response says about you.

"Dr. Lewis Thomas described medicine as "The Youngest Science" because insightful discoveries in basic research have led to the revolutionary innovations in clinical therapy that have improved the quality of life."

"One day you will read in the National Geographic of a faraway place with no smelly lousy traffic. In the green pastured mountains of Fotta-fa-Zee, everybody feels fine at a hundred and three 'cause the air they breathe is potassium-free and because they chew nuts from the Tutt-a-Tutt Tree. This gives strength to their teeth, it gives length to their hair, and they live without doctors, with nary a care"—Dr. Seuss, You're Only Old Once.

"I love the way he makes me laugh."

Dialogue Lead

This lead takes the reader into a conversation. It can take the form of an actual dialogue between two people or simply be a snippet of personal thought, such as:

"Power ten, next stroke! Shouts the coxswain over the speaker system."

"Kathy, do you believe in las brujas?"

"Peter, the woman we're about to meet, will receive her first palliative treatment today."

"Why on Earth do you want to study in Africa?"

Fact Lead

This lead gives the reader a fact or statistic connected to the topic of your essay or simply provides a piece of information about yourself or a situation, such as:

"Every PA remembers his first patient."

"In communist Hungary in 1986, ownership of property meant certain things."

"On the corner of 168th street and Broadway in New York City, there always seems to be a line of people."

Closing Your Case

The final sentence or two of your essay is also critical. It must finish your thought or assertion, which is integral to creating a positive and memorable image. Endings are the last experience an admissions officer has with your essay, so you need to make those words and thoughts count. A standard close merely summarizes the main points you have made.

Some examples of standard closes include:

"But most of all, I know that for me to bring meaning to the years of instruction my professors and textbooks have given me, I must give back to the community. So I have chosen to do that by becoming a PA."

"As a lifelong commitment to society, the medical profession most completely encompasses my career goals and moral values."

"Reminiscing about how Mr. M pulled the brown marshmallow from his chopstick, I am thankful to my campers and students, their families, and my friends for helping me to affirm that this is the path I wish to follow."

If you have introduced a clever or unusual thought in the first paragraph, try referring to it in your conclusion. The aim is for the admissions officer to leave your essay thinking, *That was a satisfying read, and I wish there were more.*

One essayist, for example, closes with:

"The once bewildered 7-year-old at the scene of an accident now has the skills and maturity to do more than change diapers; she aspires to read the film of the broken humerus or to set the cast someday soon."

The writer's reference to the bewildered 7-year-old relates to her opening story about a car accident from her youth. This stylistic touch wraps the essay up nicely and shows that she spent time planning and structuring.

WRITING THE ESSAY

Paragraphs and Transitions

Paragraphs are the pillars of the essay—they uphold and support the structure. Each one you write should express a single thought and contain a beginning, a middle, and an end. And again, this holds whether you are writing a traditional or a creative essay.

The first sentence of every paragraph (after the first, which is called the lead) plays the vital role of transitioning. An essay without good transitions is like a series of isolated islands; the reader will struggle to get from one point to the next. Use transitions as bridges between your ideas.

As you move from one paragraph to the next, you should not have to explain your story in addition to telling it. If the transitions between paragraphs require explanation, your essay is too large in scope, or the flow is not logical. A good transition statement will straddle the line between the two paragraphs.

The transition into the final paragraph is especially critical. If it is not clear how you arrived at this last idea, you have either shoe-horned a conclusion into the outline, or your outline lacks focus. It would be best if you did not have to overthink about consciously constructing transition sentences. If the concepts in your outline follow and build on one another naturally, transitions will practically write themselves. To ensure that you are not forcing your transitions, try to refrain from using words like *however, nevertheless,* and *furthermore.*

Suppose you are having trouble transitioning between paragraphs or are trying to force a transition on to a paragraph that has already been written. In that case, it may be indicative of a problem with your structure. If you suspect this to be the case, go back to your original outline and make sure that you have assigned only one point to each paragraph and that each point naturally follows the preceding one and leads to a logical conclusion. This may result in a kind of *back-to-the-drawing board* restructuring, but try not to get frustrated. This happens to even the most seasoned writers and is a normal part of the writing process.

Word Choice

Well-structured outlines, paragraphs, and transitions are essential parts of a solid essay. But the structure isn't everything. An essay can be very well organized with balanced paragraphs and smooth transitions and still come across as dull and uninspired. The most important thing you can do to make your essay more interesting is to add lots of colorful details about your life. The second most important thing you can do is pay attention to word choice.

Rule #1: Put your thesaurus away. Using a thesaurus won't make you look more intelligent; it will only make you look like you are trying to look more intelligent.

Rule #2: Focus on verbs. Keep adjectives to a minimum. Pumping your sentences full of adjectives and adverbs is not the same thing as adding detail or color. Adjectives and adverbs add a description, but verbs add action—and action is always more interesting than description.

One of the admissions officers on our panel advises using the following test to gauge the strength of your word choice.

The Verb Test

Choose a paragraph from your essay and make a list of every verb you have used. Then, compare your list to the one given in Table 6.2.

These are lists of the first 10 verbs found in 2 essays in my database. The correlation between solid verbs and high scores is undeniable. Think of it this way: if you had to choose an essay based solely on the verb list, which one would you prefer to read?

Sentence Length and Structure

Another way to analyze the strength of your writing is to examine the pacing of your sentences. To appreciate the pacing of your essay, read your essay out loud. As you read, listen to the rhythm of the sentences. Are they all the same length? If each of your sentences twists and turns for an entire paragraph, try breaking them up for variety. Remember that short sentences have a significant impact.

Table 6.2. List of Verbs

Column 1	Column 2
Said	Has met
Contorted	Can say
Complain	Know
Learned	Are usually
Spreading	May have heard
Sprang	Are
Strained	Is
Gripped	Strive
Had been living	May not be involved
Had attended	Try to perform

One way to determine if you are using various sentence lengths is to put S, M, or L (for short, medium, and long) above each sentence in a paragraph. A dull paragraph can look something like this:

M M M L M S S S M L

On the other hand, an exciting paragraph may look more like this:

S L M M L S

FINAL TOUCHES

Writing is not a one-time act. Writing is a process, and memorable writing comes from rewriting the first draft. By rewriting, you will improve your essay—guaranteed. There is no perfect amount of drafts that will ensure a great essay, but you will eventually reach a point when the thoughts of others reinforce your confidence in the strength of your writing. If you skimp on the rewriting process, you significantly reduce the chances that your essay will be as good as it could be. Don't take that chance. The following steps show you how to take your essay from rough to remarkable.

Take a Break!

You have made it through the first draft, and you deserve a reward for your hard work. However, before you do anything else—take a break! Let it sit for a couple of days. You need to distance yourself from the piece so you can gain objectivity. Writing can be an emotional and exhausting process, particularly when you write about yourself and your experiences. After you finish your first draft, you may think a bit too highly of your efforts—or you may be too harsh. Both extremes are probably inaccurate. Once you have let your work sit for a while, you will be better able to take the following (and final!) step—proofreading.

Revise

Once you have taken a break away from your essay, come back and read it through once with a fresh perspective. Analyze it as objectively as possible based on the following three components: substance, structure, and interest. Do not worry yet about surface errors and spelling mistakes; focus instead on the larger issues. Be prepared to find some significant problems with your essays and be willing to address them even though it might mean significantly more work. Also, if you find yourself unable to iron out the bugs that turn up, you should be willing to consider starting one or two of your essays from scratch, potentially with a new topic.

Use the following checklist to critique the various parts of your essays.

Substance

Substance refers to the content of your essay and the message you are sending out. It can be tough to gauge in your writing. One good way to make sure that you are saying what you think you are saying is to briefly write down your message's general idea, and in your own words. Then remove the introduction and the conclusion from your essay and have an objective reader review what is left and do the same. Finally, compare the two statements to see how similar they are. This can be especially helpful if you write a narrative to ensure that you communicate your points in the story.

Here are some questions to ask regarding content:

- Have you answered the question asked?
- Is each point that you make backed up by an example?

- Are your examples concrete and personal?
- Have you been specific? Go on a generalities hunt. Turn the generalities into specifics.
- Is the essay about you? (The answers should be *Yes!*)
- What does it say about you? Try making a list of all the words you have used to describe yourself (directly or indirectly). Does the list accurately represent you?
- Does the writing sound like you? Is it personal and informal rather than uptight or stiff?
- Read your introduction. Is it personal and written in your voice? If it is general or makes many broad claims, then have someone proofread your essay once without it. Did they notice that it was missing? If the essay can stand on its own without it, then consider removing it permanently.

Structure

To check the overall structure of your essay, do a first-sentence check. Write down the first sentence in every paragraph in order: Read through each sentence one after another and ask yourself the following:

- Would someone who was only reading these sentences still understand what you are trying to say?
- Are all your main points addressed in the first sentences?
- Do the thoughts flow naturally, or do they seem to skip around or come out of left field?

Now go back to your essay as a whole and ask yourself these questions:

- Does each paragraph stick to the thought introduced in the first sentence?
- Is each point supported by a piece of evidence?
- Are all of the paragraphs roughly the same length? When you step back and squint at your essay, do they look balanced on the page? If one is significantly longer than the rest, you are probably trying to squeeze more than one thought into it.
- Does your conclusion draw naturally from the previous paragraphs?
- Have you varied the length and structure of your sentences?

Interest

Many people think only of mechanics when they revise and rewrite their compositions. But as we know, the interest factor is crucial in keeping the admissions officers reading and making your essay memorable. Look at your essay with the interest equation in mind: personal + specific = engaging. Answer the following:

- Is the opening paragraph personal? Do you start with action or an image?
- At what point does your essay begin? Try to delete all the sentences before that point.
- Does the essay *show* rather than *tell?* Use details whenever possible to create images.
- Did you use any words that you wouldn't use in a conversation? Did you take any words from a thesaurus? (If either answer is yes, get rid of them.)
- Have you used an active voice?
- Did you do the *verb check*? Are your verbs active and exciting?
- Have you overused adjectives and adverbs?
- Have you eliminated trite expressions and clichés?
- Does it sound interesting to you? If it bores you, it will bore others.
- Will the ending give the reader a sense of completeness? For example, does the last sentence sound like the concluding sentence?

The Hunt for Red Flags

How can you know if you are writing in a passive or active voice? Certain words and phrases are red flags for passive voice, and relying on them too heavily will considerably weaken an otherwise good essay. To find out if your essay suffers from passivity, go on a hunt for all of the following, highlighting each one as you find it (Table 6.3).

When you finish, notice how much of your essay you highlighted. You do not need to eliminate these phrases, but ask yourself if each one is necessary. Then, try replacing the weak phrases with stronger ones.

Proofread

When you are satisfied with the structure and content of your essay, it's time to check for grammar, spelling, typos, and the like. There will be

Table 6.3. Passive Voice

Really	I hope	For instance
There is	Maybe	Very
It is essential that	Usually	In fact
Nonetheless/ nevertheless	Have had	I believe
In conclusion	Rather	Can be
Yet	It is important to note that	Perhaps
Although	However	May/May not
I feel	In addition	Somewhat

obvious things you can fix right away: a misspelled or misused word, a seemingly endless sentence, or improper punctuation. Keep rewriting until your words say what you want them to say. Ask yourselves these questions:

- Did I punctuate correctly?
- Did I eliminate exclamation points (except in dialogue)?
- Did I use capitalization clearly and consistently?
- Do the subjects agree in number with the verbs?
- Did I place the periods and commas inside the quotation marks?
- Do I keep contractions to a minimum? Are apostrophes in the right places?
- Did I insert the name of the right school for each new application?

Read Out Loud

To help you polish the essay even further, read it out loud. You will be amazed at the faulty grammar and awkward language that your ears can detect. It will also give you a good sense of the essay's flow and alert you to anything that sounds too abrupt or out of place. Good writing, like much music, has a certain rhythm. So how does your essay sound? Interesting and varied, or drawn out and monotonous? Reading your essay aloud is also an excellent way to catch errors that your eyes might otherwise skim over while reading silently.

ALWAYS Get Feedback!

I've mentioned this point many times throughout this chapter, but I can't emphasize enough: get Feedback! Not only will it help you see your essay objectively, as others will see it, but it is also an excellent way to get reinspired when you feel yourself burning out.

You should have already found someone to proofread for general style, structure, and content. If you have to write multiple essays for one school, you should also have evaluated the set as a whole. Now, as the final step before submitting your application, find someone new to proofread for the surface errors that only a fresh set of eyes may see. Copy this page and have them check off the questions as they proofread.

And, as we said earlier, if you are having trouble finding someone willing (and able) to dedicate the time and thought that you need to make this step effective, you may want to consider getting a professional evaluation. IvyEssays (Ivyessays.com) offers several different *editing services*. So whether you are looking for *quick Feedback or a full edit*, they have an option for you.

FUNNY MISTAKES

(AKA: See what happens when you don't proofread)

You would be amazed at what gets written into admissions essays—even at the top schools. The following is a list of some of the funniest mistakes found by the admissions officers. However, remember that behind the hilarity of these errors lurks a serious message: always proofread your essays! Otherwise, you will get the same reaction that these other applicants did: "It makes you wonder if these kids care about their essays at all," said one staff member. "I never know whether to call it apathy or ignorance," said another. But then again, at least they laugh!

- "Mt. Elgon National Park is well known for its rich deposits of herds of elephants."
- "I enjoyed my bondage with the family and especially their mule, Jake."
- "The book was very entertaining, even though it was about a dull subject, World War II."

- "I would love to attend a college where the foundation was built upon women."
- "The worst experience that I have probably ever had to go through emotionally was when other members of PETA (People for the Ethical Treatment of Animals) and I went to Pennsylvania for their annual pigeon shoot. "
- "He was a modest man with an unbelievable ego."
- "Scuba One members are volunteers, but that never stops them from trying to save someone's life."
- "Hemmingway includes no modern terminology in a *Farewell to Arms*. This, of course, is because it was not written recently."
- "I am proud to say I have sustained from the use of drugs, alcohol, and tobacco products."
- "I've been a strong advocate of the abomination of drunk driving."
- "If Homer's primary view of mortal life could be expressed in a word it would be this: life is fleeting."
- "Such things as divorces, separations, and annulments significantly reduce the need for adultery to be committed."
- "It is rewarding to hear when some of these prisoners I have fought for are released, yet triumphant when others are executed."
- "Playing the saxophone lets me develop techniques and skills to help me since I would like to become a PA."
- "However, many students would not be able to emerge from the same situation unscrewed."
- "I look at each stage as a challenge, an adventure, and another experience on my step ladder of life."
- "Bare your cross, something I have heard all my life."
- "There was one man in particular who caught my attention. He was a tiny man with ridiculously features all of which, except for his nose, seemed to drown in the mass of the delicate transparent pinkish flesh that cascaded from his forehead and flowed over the collar of his tuxedo and the edge of his bow tie."
- "Take Wordsworth, for example; every one of his words is worth a hundred words."

- "For almost all involved in these stories, premature burial has a negative effect on their lives."
- "I know that as we age, we tend to forget the bricklayers of our lives."
- "I would like to see my own ignorance wither into enlightenment."
- "Another activity I take personally is my church Youth Group."
- "The outdoors is two-dimensional, challenging my physical and mental capabilities."
- "Going to school in your wonderfully gothic setting would be an exciting challenge."
- "My mother worked hard to provide me with whatever I needed in my life, a good home, a fairly stale family and wonderful education."
- "I hope to provide in turn, a self-motivated, confident, and capable individual to add to the reputation of Quinipiac University, whose name stands up for itself. [Note: the correct spelling is Quinnipiac.]"
- "Filled with Victorian furniture and beautiful antique fixtures, even at that age, I was amazed."
- "They eagerly and happily took our bags, welcomed us in English, and quickly drove us out of the airport."
- "Do I shake the hand that has constantly bitten me?"
- "In the spring, people were literally exploding outside."
- "Freedom of speech is the ointment that sets us free."
- "I first was exposed through a friend who attends [school]."
- "As an extra, we even saw Elizabeth Taylor's home, which had a bridge attaching it to the hoe across the street."
- "*Name of Activity:* Cook and serve homeless"
- On a transcript: *AP English*
- Misspelled abbreviation on another transcript: *COMP CRAP (computer graphics)*
- Handwritten on an interview form under Academic Interests: *Writing.*

CHAPTER 7

The Interview (Part One): It's not about You; It's about Them

*C*ongratulations! You've made it to the interview phase of the physician assistant (PA) school application process, and your chances of getting accepted have increased dramatically. A typical PA program receives a thousand or more applications for a precious 25 to 50 slots each cycle. Your chance of acceptance at this point is roughly 2.5% to 5% for any given program. Many programs invite approximately 200 applicants to interview. If you make it to the interview, your chances increase to 12.5% to 25%; much better odds. Your job now is to claim your seat in the upcoming class by being the most prepared applicant in the room that day. You've taken control of your situation, and rather than be one of the thousand faceless drones trying to break into the PA profession; you've decided to do more ... be more! At last, you're not just making positive steps in the way you interview; you're making positive steps toward getting accepted!

So go ahead and pat yourself on the back, you've worked hard to get here, and you deserve to be very proud of yourself. Getting an offer to interview is just the beginning; however, not the end. You now have to take all of the knowledge and expertise I provide you and reduce it into a condensed, manageable format within the framework of the questions and answers on interview day. You may feel a bit anxious and overwhelmed at this point. But, trust me, I'm going to break all of the knowledge I present in this chapter into easy-to-digest, bite-sized nuggets of valuable information that will make you the perfect PA school applicant.

Coming into the home stretch, I'll show you how to supercharge your entire interview using targeted answers to questions you will encounter during a PA school interview. You will discover how to use the PA program's various web properties (program website, Facebook, YouTube, blogs, etc.) to uncover the qualities and multipliers (more on this later) that will set you apart from everyone else. Research is an essential part of my tailoring method, and ultimately the technique has helped me become the pioneer in coaching thousands of PA school applicants to success.

I will teach you how to infuse these qualities into your answers to tailor your responses to the program(s) where you interview. In this chapter, I'm going to take you to another level. A level that only the *perfect applicants* can reach. I will be referring to the *perfect applicant* a lot in this chapter.

Would you please think of the PA school interview process similar to studying for a test in school? To pass the test, you need to learn the material. Imagine knowing the answers to the questions on that test before taking it? Well, I'm going to provide you with the questions and answers. And not just carbon-copy answers. I will show you how to tailor your responses to the specific PA program(s) where you interview. This book is the secret weapon you need to blow away the competition and get accepted into the PA school of your choice.

In this chapter, I've compiled the most commonly asked questions that you may be asked, along with examples of *qualities* and *multipliers* that you can use to supercharge your responses. *The answers to the questions I provide are only examples, not to be memorized verbatim.* You will need to do the work and dig deep to find the qualities and multipliers for each program you interview with to find out what they value most. Additionally, the answers I supply are just suggestions. The answers I provide are excellent answers with my proven methodology behind them, helping to guide them to be solid answers that the admissions committee (ADCOM) will want to hear. Still, they're not necessarily 100% the correct answers for you. My formula is a guide; use it to mold your answers based on personal experiences, qualities, and values. Don't memorize the replies in this chapter; you will come off as fake and unnatural at your interview. Instead, use this chapter as a springboard to help you rise above the competition and make a favorable impression on the ADCOM.

In addition to samples of the most common questions and answers, I'm also providing you with the most common DOS and DON'TS for each question, which will give you some additional insight and make answering the question much more effortless.

Remember it's tailoring the interview to the program(s) you are interviewing with that is the most important thing.

BEFORE THE INTERVIEW

Okay, hopefully, you're pumped up thinking about how much you're going to learn in this chapter; it's now time to go to work! I'm going to break this section down into five easy-to-manage segments.

Okay, let's get started!

General Preparation

You've done all of the work necessary to get your CASPA application completed and submitted. You wait in anticipation to hear back from the PA programs you applied to, and then one day, you open your email and see that your top choice PA program has sent you a response. You hold your breath, your heart starts pounding, and you quickly click to open it up. You read, "Congratulations, we would like to extend you an offer to interview at our PA program." After you jump up and down, call your friends, and soak up the moment, it's now time to prepare for the final and most challenging piece of the PA school application process. Your job has just begun.

You should be very proud of yourself for a job well done. Go out and celebrate, then be ready to come back and do the work of preparing for your PA school interview.

You look great on paper, but now it's time to prepare to show the ADCOM that you look the part in person too. That means you must begin preparing for your interview long before you stand tall before the ADCOM.

The sooner you complete the work, the sooner you can review these example questions and answers and prepare your responses. So don't procrastinate; get it done ASAP!

Sleep Hygiene

If you are used to keeping irregular hours, going out with your friends too late in the morning, or just not getting the recommended 8 hours of sleep per night, now is the time to get on a regular sleep schedule. Getting enough sleep enables you to be fresh every day and have the energy to do the upcoming work necessary to perform your best on the day of your interview.

Take Care of Yourself

If you don't already exercise, start slowly with an exercise routine that will energize you daily. What is the best exercise? The one you'll do! Cut back on your caffeine use. At this point, you should be on a natural "high" anyway. Start eating a healthy diet, low in sugar and high in protein. Get your body running like a well-oiled machine, and by the time your interview comes, you'll be happy, healthy, and confident.

The night before the interview, be sure to arrive at your hotel early (if you're traveling). I strongly recommend that you do a *dry run* and walk or drive to the exact location of the building and room where you will be interviewing the next day. Check out the traffic conditions and the length of time it will take you to get there. Anticipate the worst-case scenario, and leave early in the morning. You can always go to a restaurant for a small breakfast if you have a lot of spare time. Don't forget to carry the program's phone number, just in case you hit a traffic jam or for some unforeseen reason, and you will be late.

Be sure to eat well the night before your interview. Have a light dinner, and don't eat anything that may linger on your breath. Also, don't drink alcohol that night. You certainly don't want to smell like you just came from the bar before your interview.

Take out your suit (yes, wear a suit!), shirt/blouse, belt, socks, and shoes. Try everything on BEFORE the interview. Make sure everything looks impeccable, shoes shined, no stains on your clothes, and place everything in a space where you don't have to go searching for any items in the morning. You will be nervous enough, and you don't need to be frantically searching for your belt for 15 minutes on the morning of your interview.

Next, take 15 to 20 minutes to sit quietly in your room. Close your eyes, and visualize your entire interview. See yourself impeccably dressed, confident, answering all of the interview questions with ease. This technique is powerful, and many professional athletes use it before a big game. For example, a basketball player may visualize herself making every shot she takes, stealing the ball on defense, and grabbing rebound after rebound. Visualization is the equivalent of doing a dry run in your mind.

I always advise bringing a small mirror with you to the interview. You may want to look closely at your face, teeth, hair, etc., immediately before entering the interview room. Sometimes PA programs offer food and drinks during the day. Having mustard on your face or a piece of broccoli caught between your teeth will certainly not score you any points. And believe me, I've seen it all.

The Day of the Interview

Set your alarm clock to go off early, and ask the hotel front desk to provide you with a wake-up call as a backup. Have a small breakfast before getting dressed. Take a good look in the mirror, and keep your jacket on a hanger while traveling to the interview. Be sure to recheck yourself in the bathroom mirror once you're ready to go. Do not overdo the perfume or cologne, and please, no nose rings, tongue rings, or bright pink hair. Now is not the time to *express yourself.*

I recommend that you arrive at least 15 minutes early; no sooner, no later. If you are very early, sit in the car or a restaurant, and practice your answers to the questions. Some applicants like to meditate to calm their nerves. Others want to make phone calls to some of their friends or a significant other to get moral support.

DO NOT bring a cell phone into your interview. You will be too tempted to check text messages or perhaps sneak in a phone call. Even worse, you don't want your cell phone to ring (or vibrate) in the middle of your interview.

Be sure to greet everyone you encounter at the program with a smile and a handshake. If you say the wrong thing to the receptionist, she will likely pass on this negative experience to one of the committee members she works with every day, which will not help your chances. So be friendly, and smile at everyone.

Silence Your Inner Critic

When you walk into your interview and meet the other applicants (the *competition*), your inner critic inside of your brain may go to work. "I'm not good enough; The other applicants are more qualified than I am; I don't belong here." The inner critic can be your worst enemy in this situation, and you need to know how to silence it. A straightforward technique is to say *Stop* in your mind each time a negative thought enters it. Do this 20 times if you have to. Eventually, the negative thoughts will quiet down, and you'll be able to focus on the task at hand. I will teach you a technique to help you with anxiety later in the chapter.

Think about the fact that you would not be here if you didn't have what it takes. The ADCOM screened your application, and they selected you for an interview. You have what it takes, so focus on that. Everybody in that room has an equal chance. However, if you use the *quality* and *multiplier* techniques I show you, you will be much more prepared than anyone else.

Additionally, when you walk in and meet the other applicants, be the first to extend a handshake and introduce yourself. If an applicant walks in after you arrive, do the same. Do not allow yourself to be intimidated by the applicant who will boast about his medical experience or GPA. Keep the conversations light and cursory. If necessary, walk into a quiet corner and focus on the task at hand.

Types of Interviews

Many of you will have no idea what to expect when showing up for your PA school interview. I'm not just talking about the questions and answers; I'm talking about the various interview formats you may encounter during this critical phase of the application process. Each program utilizes a structure to assess you as an applicant. The design depends on what values and qualities they seek from their ideal applicants. It would help if you prepared for each of these formats to give a peak performance. Let's take a look at the most common forms that you may encounter.

The Solo Interview

The one-on-one interview is the traditional interview format. A high-level program faculty member typically conducts your solo interview. This member will have a critical role in the decision-making process, so you must be at the top of your game. **The solo interviewer will have a crucial set of qualities and traits that she is looking for, and this is your chance to show her how perfectly you match her criteria.** Once you finish reading this chapter, you will feel very comfortable in this traditional interview format. Before you know it, you'll be visualizing your seat in the classroom. The best way to do this is to follow the steps I've laid out for you in this chapter with perfectly tailored answers (more on this later).

The Panel Interview

Imagine walking through the door, and there are three smiling faces staring back at you (or maybe not smiling?). This interview format is certainly a bit more anxiety-provoking, but not to worry. There are several reasons why a program uses the panel interview format, but the main reason is to eliminate any bias that one interviewer may have toward an applicant. It also ramps up the pressure a little bit on the applicant, allowing the interviewers to see how well you handle stress and deal with authority.

To relieve some pressure and prepare for this interview format, try to find out beforehand if a panel interview is on the agenda, how many people will be on the panel, and get their names. If the program provides the interviewers' names, do some research and find out as much information about each member. Perhaps one won a specific award or was past president of the American Academy of Physician Assistants (AAPA). Maybe you went to the same college as one of the members, or you both played the same sport. Also, be prepared for the panel to change members on you. Perhaps the three people you've researched interviewed with the first applicant of the day, but the panel switches out with three other members for *your* panel interview. Don't panic! As long as you've read this book and prepared your answers to the most common questions, you'll be fine.

One suggestion I have—no, one strong recommendation—is to make eye contact with each member on the panel. I recommend maintaining eye contact with *each* of them for approximately 5 seconds at a time. Repeat this process until you've fully answered the question. Engaging everyone at the table or risk alienating committee members who may develop a subconscious resentment toward you is imperative. (More on this in the next chapter.)

One applicant told me that she was in a panel interview, and one of the interviewers got up in the middle of the session, took a seat behind her, and started asking her questions from a position behind her back. Perhaps this is a technique to see how you handle stress. If this happens to you, remember that eye contact is the key to gaining credibility and trust. So turn your chair *sideways and look to your left or right to* establish eye contact with everyone.

The Multiple Applicant Interview

In my opinion, this is one of the most stressful interviews you will face. You're sitting in a room with other applicants who want *your* seat in the program. Don't worry; I'm going to give you some sure-fire techniques to help ensure your voice stands out from the crowd in a good way. The multiple applicant interview is an excellent opportunity to showcase your ability to interact well with others and allow the committee to see if you'd be a good *fit* for their program. The multiple applicants' interviews will work to your benefit if you prepare. Think about it, you'll be in a room full of applicants that aren't using qualities and multipliers as part of their responses, and you will undoubtedly stand out from the rest of the applicants.

PA programs value teamwork; it's necessary if a class will gel and help each other through an intense PA program. This type of interview is an excellent way for the members to see if they *play well with others*. Are you going to be a team player willing to help others or a loner who can't be bothered by students who may be having difficulties? This group interview is not a time to be passive or shy. You want to be assertive but not aggressive. The multiple applicants' interviews should create a win-win situation. Be balanced in your approach to this type of interview. You don't want to be the person who says nothing and appears to be intimated by the other applicants.

On the other hand, you don't want to be the aggressive, chatty, know-it-all who thinks he will score high by dominating the competition and not allowing them the time to speak. If you want to ace the multiple applicant interview, show your leadership skills by knowing when to speak and listen. If someone answers a question, perhaps you can interject by saying, "I think Sally makes a good point, and I might add …" Do not use the word *but,* because it implies you disagree with Sally.

The Multiple Mini-Interview (MMI)

Multiple mini-interviews (MMIs) consist of a series of short, structured interview stations used to assess non-cognitive qualities, including cultural sensitivity, maturity, teamwork, empathy, reliability, and communication skills.

Before starting each mini-interview rotation, candidates receive a question/scenario and have a designated period to prepare an answer. For instance, there may be a prompt on the door outside of the room. You may have 3 minutes to read the prompt, then enter the room and have 7 minutes to provide your answer.

Upon entering the interview room, the candidate has a short exchange with an interviewer/assessor. In some situations, the interviewer observes while the action takes place between the applicant and an actor.

At the end of each mini-interview, the interviewer evaluates the candidate's performance while the applicant moves to the next station. This pattern repeats itself for several stations. The questions asked are usually situational questions that touch on the following:

- Ethical decision making
- Critical thinking
- Communication skills
- Current health care and societal issues

Although participants must relate to the scenario posed at each station, it is essential to note that the MMI doesn't necessarily test specific knowledge in the field. Instead, the interviewers evaluate each candidate's thought process and ability to think on one's feet. As such, there are no right or wrong answers. Each applicant should look at the question from a variety of perspectives.

I provide a chapter dedicated to the MMI in the next section.

The Student Interview

The student interview usually consists of two or three first- or second-year students, asking you questions in a more relaxed format. But don't be fooled by the conversational nature of this interview. The students will have a say on whether they like you or not, particularly evaluating you as someone they would like to have as a classmate. **So treat the students with the utmost respect. Look at this interview as an excellent opportunity to tell them why you should attend their program.**

You are not likely to be asked traditional interview questions in the student interview. Still, if you've followed the guidance in this book, you'll be prepared to discuss qualities and multipliers that you've researched before the interview. Be sure to visit the student society website or blog to find out what special events or projects they find meaningful. Students are very proud of their program and their chosen events. Perhaps a group of students went on a mission trip to South America to provide vaccinations to children in isolated regions of a country. It would be nice to know this information ahead of time. Take the time to do your homework and let the students know that you have the same values and qualities as they have.

Dos and Don'ts for the PA School Interview

Now that you know how to prepare for the various PA school interviews you may encounter, let's take a list of DOS and DON'TS.

Do your homework (research). Learn everything you can about the program(s) where you will be interviewing. Start early. The program's website is the first place to start. Leave no stone unturned. View every page and link on the site. Don't forget about social media, either. Check out the program on Facebook, Google, Blogs, Student sites, and YouTube.

How many applicants do you think will know about this effort come interview day? Can you infuse these qualities into some of your answers to interview questions at Barry? Underlined are the *qualities*, and the *multiplier* is the Event (No More Tears Charity Golf Tournament).

DON'T: Continuously call the program and become a nuisance. Don't ask questions that you should know from searching the program's website.

DO: Invest in a new suit if you don't have one or rent one if necessary. The point is, always lean toward overdressing rather than under-dressing.

DON'T: Come to the interview with nose rings, tongue rings, flashy jewelry, low-cut blouses, unkempt hair, or a wrinkled outfit. Dress for success. You want the focus to be on you and not your attire.

DO: Eat a simple, well-balanced meal the night before your interview. Also, be sure to eat a good breakfast in the morning before the interview.

DON'T: Eat a bunch of spicy food, or junk food, the night before your interview. You don't want to have acid reflux first thing in the morning, making you feel miserable. Also, do not drink alcohol before your interview to calm your nerves. I will teach you a much better way to deal with anxiety later in the chapter.

DO: Get a good night's sleep the night before.

DON'T: Stay up all night stressing over the interview or cramming information into your brain. Instead, rest assured you've done the work. Perhaps watch a movie, and relax as best you can.

DO: Take a shower, brush your teeth, and spend the time to look your best. As you'll see in the next chapter, the visual component of an interview will weigh significantly on your score.

DON'T: Smoke before your interview; your clothes will smell like tobacco, and being a smoker is not the best way to show that you advocate for health.

DO: Arrive early for your interview, review your notes, and practice the anxiety-relieving technique that I will teach you in the next section.

DON'T: Be rude to *anyone* you meet at the program, including the other applicants. For example, if the receptionist asks you, "Did you have any trouble finding us?," your response should be: "Absolutely not, you gave excellent directions, thank you." You want to start things off on a positive note.

DO: Be a natural person. In other words, do your best to be likable, trustworthy, and credible.

DON'T: Panic. Remember, *it's not about you; it's about them.* So get out of your head and shut off that inner critic. You prepared for this interview. Remember that the committee wants you to solve their problem—finding the perfect applicant with all of the qualities *they* seek.

In this next section, I will share a technique to quiet your mind and relieve the anxiety that you are likely to feel on the day of your interview.

Dealing with Anxiety

As soon as you open your eyes on the morning of your interview, I can assure you that your heart will start racing, your breath will be shallow and rapid, and you will probably have a knot in the pit of your stomach. Don't panic! What you're experiencing is healthy anxiety. Your body's physiology is acting appropriately. The challenge is to avoid panicking.

For example, think about the following situation: You come out of your friend's house and begin walking to your car. You suddenly hear the loud barking of a giant dog, foaming at the mouth and making a B-line right toward you. As a result, your physiology begins to go into fight-or-flight mode; your pupils immediately dilate, your breathing becomes rapid and shallow, and your heart rate goes through the roof. I think it's safe to say that it's not exactly the best moment to figure out your taxes at a time like this. So if you want to be able to think, particularly on the day of your interview, you need to control your physiology because you're likely to be in fight-or-flight mode when you enter the building.

The day of your interview is not a time to *wing it!* If so, your plan will cause a lot more anxiety, and you will be in the fight-or-flight mode throughout the entire interview process. In addition, you will have a tough time answering interview questions if you can't change this physiological response quickly.

The SHIELD Technique

Dr. Eva Selhub, a mind/body expert, resiliency coach, motivational speaker, and executive coach, teaches a powerful technique to reduce a person's stress and anxiety instantly. Her approach is to put up your SHIELD. While waiting to be called into the room, you can use this technique, and nobody will have to know that you're using it.

The acronym stands for:

Stop
Honor the feeling
Inhale
Exhale
Listen
Decide

Author of *The Love Response*, Dr. Selhub promotes a simple philosophy: At its best, stress motivates. At its worst, stress annihilates. Good leaders motivate. Bad leaders annihilate.

The choice is yours to decide how stress will influence your leadership.

If you find yourself in an anxiety-provoking or stressful situation (like the PA school interview), you can instantly use the SHIELD™ technique to change your physiology.

As a result, if you utilize this technique, your breathing will slow down, your heart rate will decrease, your pupils will return to normal size, and you will be able to think much more clearly.

Here is how the technique works:

> Once you feel your anxiety level becoming too high, *stop* what you are doing. Then, ***honor the feeling***. Ask yourself: are you anxious, afraid, frustrated, angry, lonely, or tired? Next, *inhale* and *exhale* 10 times in a row. (When you breathe in, imagine filling an empty balloon in your belly with your breath. When you breathe out, imagine deflating the balloon). Repeat the breaths 10 times, and you will notice a soothing, calming effect. By this time, your adrenaline is dropping, and you will think clearly and focus on the task at hand. So, ***listen*** to your mind and become aware of your thoughts and feelings now. Finally, ***decide*** to do something different than ruminating, which is counterproductive. Now, your body is out of fight-or-flight mode.

You can repeat the above technique as many times as necessary to help you relax and focus.

Silencing the Inner Critic

In a variety of stressful situations, we become our own worst enemy. I can remember arriving for my interview at Yale and meeting all of my *competition*. Everyone in the room had a master's degree, except for me. My inner critic came alive; *I'm never going to get in!* I was very hard on myself and highly judgmental. Negative self-talk only serves to perpetuate the anxiety and make things worse.

Here are some things *your* inner critic may shout at you on the day of your interview:

- *I should have prepared more.*
- *Everyone here is more qualified than I am.*
- *I'll never get accepted.*
- *I'm a loser; I don't belong here.*
- *I'm going to blow this interview.*

Don't wait until your interview to address your inner critic. Here are some steps that you can take to deal with your internal critic weeks or months before your interview:

1. *Monitor your thoughts.*

   Becoming aware of your inner critic's voice—if you will—is the first step. You can achieve this by simply being mindful of those thoughts. Just notice when and where the thoughts occur, and then write them down on a piece of paper or in a journal.

   You may become acutely aware of specific patterns in your thinking. Once you master being mindful and get the negative thoughts on paper, you can silence the inner critic.

2. *Notice your judgments.*

   Instead of making judgments, try describing your thoughts or feelings. For example, you may be having a conversation with a fellow student about a class you are both taking. You may like the professor, and in the course of the conversation, you might say, *Professor Jones is a great teacher.* On the other hand, your classmate might disagree with you and state; *I think he's a terrible teacher.* Both of you are making judgments and probably putting the other person on guard to defend their decision.

   If you said instead, *I appreciate that Professor Jones always comes prepared to class. It makes it easier for me to stay focused.*

But, again, you are not judgmental; you are simply describing the way you *feel* about him. Nobody can dispute that, not even your friend.

The point is that when we are judgmental, especially of ourselves, we promote more intense feelings of negativity. And at the interview, we want to stay positive.

3. *Challenge your automatic negative thoughts.*

Feelings aren't facts! Once you practice mindfulness and become good at documenting your thoughts (judgments), it is time to challenge those negative thoughts with the facts. You may feel like you don't have what it takes to be accepted, but you may change your mind if you look at the facts.

For example, if you were to review your CASPA application, you would see that you've worked hard to complete the requirements for PA school. The fact that you received an offer to interview means that you've already beat out several hundred applicants to get the interview. So although you may certainly feel like you don't have what it takes to get accepted, the facts prove otherwise.

Try to challenge all of your negative thoughts with the facts. Chances are, you will find that you are beating yourself up for no reason.

4. *Practice, not perfection.*

The goal of practicing mindfulness and keeping your judgments in check is to achieve awareness and make gradual changes. Becoming aware of the problem is the first step. However, if you are in denial about how your judgments and negative thoughts affect your mindset, you will not be able to make any progress at all. It takes constant vigilance to achieve improvement by being mindful.

5. *Reevaluate your values.*

Make sure that whatever you are beating yourself up over is worth achieving. Some goals, like kindness, integrity, and self-discipline, enhance the meaning and quality of life. Some goals only feed into your sense of defectiveness. Some people think, *If I only went to a better school, I'd have more self-esteem.* By the way, the best way to increase self-esteem is to do esteemable things!

Final Preparation

Remember, your objective at the interview is to help the interviewers' job become a little easier by showing them that you have the qualities and values they're looking for in a perfect applicant. Remember my mantra; *It's not about you; it's about them.* Your interviewer is not out to trip you up. He's a regular person, with a family, worries, and insecurities just like you. He may be just as nervous as you are.

Be prepared for multiple interviews. I recommend that you call the program beforehand to see if they will tell you how many interviews you will have, and perhaps even who will be your interviewers. Find out if they use traditional questions, behavioral questions, or an MMI format. Furthermore, ask if the interview is an *open* interview or a *closed* interview. An *open* interview means the committee members have access to your CASPA application during the interview. A *closed* interview means the committee members don't have access to your CASPA application and likely know nothing about you or your qualifications.

Evaluations begin from the time you enter the building until the time you exit the building. Maintain a professional appearance and persona throughout the entire process. Greet everyone with a smile and a handshake and take no one for granted. Remember that although you may only be there for one day, these people spend 40 hours a week together, just like in any other job. They're like a small family, and they've seen a lot of candidates come and go. If you say something negative or controversial in front of the receptionist, don't be surprised if she passes that information to the committee members. You've done too much work to be here, and it would be a tragedy to get rejected because you insulted one of the staff.

Finally, be sure to treat the student interviewers with the utmost respect. Don't let your guard down because you think they don't say much about scoring your interview. Instead, take advantage of the opportunity to let them tell you what they like most about the program? As I'll mention in another section of this chapter, you want to be likable above all else.

THE TAILORING METHOD

In this next section, I'll introduce you to a powerful tool that will help you leave the competition in the dust: the tailoring method. I will also explain the idea of the *perfect applicant*. But, more importantly, I'll finally introduce the essential pieces to the "interview question puzzle," the *qualities*, and *multipliers*.

If you've read any of my books, you've probably noticed that I do things a little differently than anyone else. As the pioneer in PA school applicant coaching, and author of four books dedicated to helping PA school applicants, you know that I use specialized techniques and training to help applicants get accepted! There are many more PA school coaches available to PA school applicants now than when I started in 1996; however, none have the longevity, experience, and knowledge that I've gained over the past 20 years working with applicants from all over the country. So, yes, I help applicants get accepted!

Okay, so what is my secret? How have I been able to help so many applicants succeed? Because there is one key to success that I teach those I coach:

It's not about you; it's about them!

You may *think* it's about you. After all, you have a strong passion for becoming a PA; you've completed all of the prerequisites for PA school. In addition, you have a 3.7 science GPA, 3,000 hours of hands-on medical experience, phenomenal GRE scores, and excellent references. You're now ready to *strut your stuff* at the interview.

But it's *not* about you. It's about meeting the program's needs and demonstrating that you have everything they look for in a perfect applicant. First, of course, the interviewer(s) look to see if you have the qualities to become a great student and a great PA. But, more importantly, do you have what it takes to be a good classmate, complete the rigorous program, pass your boards, and be a respectable representative of their program out in the community?

Many other PAs, friends, coworkers, and PA school coaches will tell you that the best thing you can do at your interview is summarize *your* past experiences and highlight *your* strengths and accomplishments. And to be honest, when those strengths and experiences are better than the other applicants, it's often enough to get accepted.

In contrast, my philosophy considers the "old school" way of interviewing. What if you don't have a clear-cut advantage over the other applicants? There will be the best of the best at the interview in the considerable applicant pool, and *everyone* will have a strong resume.

The program knows exactly the type of applicant they're going to accept long before you enter the interview room. Many of the interviewers have been doing this for a long time. They instinctively know the qualities and traits the program desires. They don't know the specific name of the applicants they will accept but take my word for it, the committee members understand the type of person, and more importantly, they know the strengths (or qualities) that this person MUST possess.

The question now becomes, how do you become that person the program wants to accept? How do you demonstrate the qualities that the program values most?

You must point out ways to add value to the program: how to help them achieve their goals based on your past training and experience. Then, of course, you'll get your reward if they invite you to join the upcoming class. But be more interested in them than you are in yourself. Be there for them. Take it from my experience being on an ADCOM; it's a tough job, so help them make the right decision.

For starters, point out what you have to offer the program: how can you help them achieve their goals based upon your past training and experience?

But how does one do this?

By using the tailoring method, of course!

So, it should be clear that the program you are about to interview already knows the type of applicant they want to accept. I refer to this person as the *perfect applicant*.

The Perfect Applicant

You will see this term a lot in this chapter because my goal is to turn you into this person before entering the interview room.

What is a *perfect applicant*? As mentioned above, every program already has the kind of person in mind they want to accept into their program. Based on your research, the person will need to demonstrate at least two or three qualities the program values or emphasizes. When the program is conducting interviews, the person who best reflects these qualities is the one who is going to score the highest at the interview. This person is the perfect applicant.

Here is a simple formula to remember if you want to be the perfect applicant:

$$PA = (A + Q)^m$$

To better understand this formula, I'm going to break down the components for you.

PA = Perfect Applicant
A = Answer

Simply stated, the A in the equation is the answer you provide to the question the interviewer asks you. **Ideally, this will be a success story from your past, one that demonstrates an example of you succeeding in your past jobs or any other relevant scenarios.**

It's always a good idea to prepare for every interview with a few of these success stories at your disposal. Everyone can draw a blank when asked a question at an interview. If you have a few of these success stories to fall back on, you can avoid that awkward silence that occurs when you draw that blank.

Q = Qualities

Qualities are what make up the perfect applicant. These are generally different types of knowledge, skills, or abilities that the program considers paramount. If you want to set yourself apart in the interview, these are the things you need to reference or exemplify in your interview.

As mentioned above, the interviewer(s) will have a set of qualities in mind that the perfect applicant must have. It is your job to determine these qualities and demonstrate to the interviewer that you possess them. I'll show you how to find those qualities in the next section. I'll also show you how to infuse these qualities into your answer.

Example Qualities

Table 7.1. Example Qualities.

Accountability	Adaptability	Ability to handle stress
Assertive	Academic ability	Analytical thinking
Attention to detail	Balanced	Collaboration
Cooperation	Confidence	Compassion
Caring	Discipline	Diversity
Empathetic	Energy	Ethical
Friendly	Humility	Hard working
Knows when to ask for help	Leadership	Life-long learner
Listener	Maturity	Proactive
Problem solver	Service oriented	Strong interpersonal skills

m = multipliers

Multipliers are the *icing on the cake* in your interview, a supercharger or booster for each of your answers. Multipliers are nuggets of information that you can bring up in your interview that the interviewer is not expecting you to know. Generally speaking, this would include particular programs, initiatives or events, volunteer programs, to name a few. The *m* acts as an exponent because it increases your chance of being the perfect applicant exponentially!

Multipliers are so effective because they help you demonstrate your level of knowledge of the program and their culture and make a statement about the amount of preparation you've done.

Using multipliers can make you look like you're already a student in the interviewer's eyes.

I'm going to show you how to find multipliers in the next section.

I hope that makes sense to you as a PA school applicant. Let's again review the idea of the equation:

$$\text{Perfect Applicant} = (\text{Answer} + \text{Question})^{\text{multiplier}}$$

When the interviewer asks you a question at your PA school interview, they expect you to respond. You have a choice. You can give them a straight, literal, carbon-copy answer that is your best attempt at giving them the information they need, or you can utilize the tailoring method by using the perfect applicant principle above. First, answer your question by infusing a quality (A + Q) the program is looking for in a qualified applicant. Then, put the icing on the cake by including a multiplier (m).

The truth is your competition won't stand a chance if they are simply using the *old-school* interview techniques.

So obviously, the next question is:

How do I find the specific qualities that the program values?

Discovering these qualities is the key because you can't simply guess which qualities you *think* the program values. You have to know precisely. If you try to be clever and emphasize a quality that the program doesn't value, you're just going to sound like every vanilla applicant who interviews that day.

Our goal is to have you rise to the top of the applicant pool, so let me show you how to identify which qualities your program values, and at the same time, it will reveal how to find some of the multipliers that are like a bonus!

Finding Qualities and Multipliers

It is essential to respond to interview questions by infusing the program's desired perfect applicant qualities into your answers. The next step is to figure out what these qualities and multipliers are AND where you find them.

Preparing for the PA school interview process has changed dramatically with the proliferation of technology, namely the internet. In the old days, we had to request program brochures, attend the open house, call the program, and ask questions. The research was limited to speaking with program graduates, purchasing a hard copy of the old PA Programs Directory, printed information from the AAPA, or your state (constituent) chapter of the AAPA. The research was all cursory information available to everyone else; no *top secret* stuff. Thus, everyone walked into the interview on an even playing field.

Times have changed, however. Every PA program publishes information everywhere on the internet. With the explosion of the internet comes an explosion of information available to PA school applicants at your fingertips, and all you have to do is complete your homework and take advantage of this information.

Websites replace brochures for every program. The website's photos, videos, and other multimedia programs are now able to give prospective applicants a glimpse into their culture, mission, and values. So even before you walk into the interview room, you will have a good idea of what it will be like to attend their program.

But that's not all.

They also leave clues. What kind of clues? Hints of the sort that are very interesting to me, and from now on, will be fascinating to you. Beginning with the program's website, this is where we start to dig around for potential qualities and multipliers, the life-blood of the tailoring method, and perhaps the most influential part of a successful PA school interview.

You may be thinking, *Looking on the program's website is not exactly a revolutionary idea.* You know what? You'd be surprised how many of the applicants I coach thought the same thing at the beginning.

But it's not just about gathering some background information on the program or simply studying their mission and values before heading into your interview. When I tell you that PA programs are leaving clues on their website, I mean it. One of the absolute best places to discover the types of qualities that their perfect applicant must possess is their website, and this is how you do it.

1. General Information

Begin by going to the program's website and **get a good feel for all of the available general information**, including:

- History of the program
- Longevity of the program
- First-time pass/fail rates on the PANCE
- Location
- Any recent news items
- Cadaver lab
- International clinical rotations
- Class size
- Learning style of the program; problem-based learning?

These are just the basics! None of this information will set you apart from your competitors, but you will surely set yourself apart (the wrong way) if you don't know this stuff inside and out. The point is you need to **get a feel for the program's culture, what they value most, any current events or volunteer work the students participate in, or any news stories relevant to the program.**

Notice any themes that may jump out at you. I have found that occasionally, qualities and multipliers can be found among the general information, depending on how much information the program chooses to present on their website. For example, you may get a sense that the program values *diversity* and *working with underserved populations*. Take note of anything the program is going out of its way to share.

2. Finding Qualities

Once you have a solid understanding of the general information, the next thing you need to do is *drill down* to get some more interview-focused information. Again, this is where social media pages, student blogs, Google, and student society pages usually come into play.

Be sure to read the *About Us* link, then check the other internet resources mentioned above. You'd be surprised to see what pops up from doing a simple Google search of the program.

Make sure to read the mission statement thoroughly. The program will usually tell you precisely what types of applicants they prefer. For example, sometimes, they look for students who come from *diverse* backgrounds. Sometimes they look for *in-state* applicants who want to stay and work in the state after graduation. Occasionally, they might publish that they are looking for applicants to work in *underserved areas* after graduating.

What does this mean for you, the interviewee? First, as I mentioned earlier in the chapter, you need to tailor your answers to your interviewing program. You do this by infusing your solutions to their questions with qualities and multipliers.

I pulled these qualities from the Duke University PA Program Home Page:

We value:

- *Diversity and inclusion*
- *Integrity*
- *Excellence*
- *Professionalism*
- *Team work and respect*
- *Kindness and compassion*
- *Scholarship*

You will notice that Duke has hinted how important it is to find applicants with diversity as their top-listed value. Therefore, you must be able to demonstrate that you possess this quality. If you cannot show this quality, pick one of the others to provide an example of how you've shown that quality.

How do you do this?

Carefully choose to infuse your answers with this quality identified above.

Now keep this in mind. A program can reveal its desired perfect applicant qualities in many different formats; videos, blog posts, Google, Facebook, and even YouTube. The point is you have to dig around to see what you can turn up. Trust me; it's in your best interest!

In the Question and Answer portion of this chapter, I'll show you examples of how to tailor your responses to the program(s) you are interviewing with using qualities.

3. Finding Multipliers

The way to find multipliers on the program's website is not unlike searching for qualities. The home page is undoubtedly the place to get started.

> *The PA Program is committed to recruiting and enrolling a wide range of students including but not limited to those who are underrepresented in the PA profession because PAs interact with patients, families, and communities from diverse backgrounds.*

The multipliers are not something that will necessarily be as obvious. Why? Well, mainly because many of the interviewers don't even know that multipliers exist. Instead, they don't expect you, the interviewee, to zone in on them like a ninja and use them as a secret weapon in your interview.

As I mentioned before, **multipliers are like the *cherry on the top* of your interview answer. Multipliers help separate you from everybody else at the interview.** So please focus on the program's upcoming (or past) events, special programs they offer, or any outreach programs or initiatives they support.

Here is a sample multiplier from a second-year PA student's blog entry at Duke.

Second-Year Student Blog: Katherine Caro

> *I appreciate Yale's PA program because of its commitment to <u>community service and helping underserved populations.</u> For example, I'm currently in my family practice rotation, and I get to visit <u>a soup kitchen</u> once per week and provide medical care to a local homeless community. We have a limited supply of medications that we pass out and treat some of the most common illnesses.*
>
> *As students, we also have many opportunities to help the local community outside of medicine. For example, I helped a local "Habitat for Humanity" group build low-cost housing.*
>
> *I also have the opportunity to do a rural medicine rotation in Kentucky. We work out of a trailer to provide <u>care to a local migrant community.</u> This program has been a part of Yale's PA program for decades. This commitment was something I noticed immediately on my interview day while learning about various opportunities afforded by the program.*

Bringing up this multiplier (*Underserved Community Scholar Program*) gives your answer a little boost. This response shows that you have done your research, but in reality, provides the interviewer with the feeling that you are *already one of them.* You bridge the gap between being an applicant and a student by showing your level of comfort and understanding of how the program does things.

Final Thought on Qualities and Multipliers

Everything said and done, finding qualities and multipliers on a program's website is not especially difficult. As long as you take the time to explore the website, making sure to *leave no stone unturned*, you will be sure to find the qualities and multipliers you need to position yourself as the perfect applicant.

However, the program's website is not the only place to reveal its qualities and multipliers. For example, Google *Emory PA Program Special Events*, and see what you find. You will find that the class of 2015 PA students is rehabilitating a home for Habitat for Humanity during orientation week, August 2013. You can replace *Emory PA Program* with any program you choose in your Google search to find tiny pearls of information.

QUESTIONS AND ANSWERS

Okay, let's get to the interview questions you may need to answer. First, I will present a few samples from each interview format to answer questions using qualities and multipliers. Then, I will provide a list of many other questions the committee will likely ask at your interview, and I will give you a blueprint to help you find and document your qualities and multipliers for each program.

Traditional Versus Behavioral Questions

Most interview questions fall into two broad categories, with some slight overlap. The two categories are traditional interview questions and *behavioral* or competency-type questions.

Traditional questions are the most commonly asked questions at a PA-school interview. They are also the easiest to prepare for since almost every PA program asks similar questions in this format.

Traditional interview questions allow the interviewer to get a feel for:

• your knowledge of the PA profession
• your reasons for choosing the PA profession
• your personality
• your seriousness as an applicant (are you just testing the water, or are you a serious candidate?)

- your communication skills
- your interpersonal skills
- your fitness for the program

There is an art and a science to conducting a great interview. A great interview goes beyond the traditional questions that one would expect and uses various techniques and styles to extract information from the candidate. As a PA, you will have to think on your feet and work under stressful conditions. The ADCOM wants to know if you have what it takes to make it through school and be a good ambassador for their program once you graduate.

More and more PA programs are utilizing a technique called *behavioral interviewing*. Interviewers can interpret what you say about yourself and your past behavior to indicate how you will behave in the future.

As you probably know from watching many crime dramas on television, someone with a history of criminal activity becomes a prime suspect; if someone broke the law before, it is statistically likely that they will do it again at some point.

You are a *prime suspect* for acceptance into the PA program's upcoming class. The committee is looking to see how you've responded to situations in the past, which can help them predict how successfully you will react to similar situations when you're a practicing PA.

It's in your best interest to be able to demonstrate through the use of recent, relevant examples that you have done similar jobs with proven success. When the interviewer begins to see patterns and hear about successes in your past experiences, you will be considered a serious candidate for admission.

Behavioral questions can catch you off guard if you are not used to them and have not prepared for them. They require a lot more thinking than traditional questions. *"How do you handle stress?* (a traditional-type question) is a lot easier to answer than *Tell me about a time when you had to endure a stressful situation?*

Because behavioral questions are a bit more expressive than traditional questions, they seem to invite you to open up and be more of a human personality to the interviewer. Remember, though, this is not a time to bear your soul.

Behavioral questions may even seem like trick questions because they definitely require you to do some thinking and might even require some soul-searching. You need to prepare ahead of time for these questions. Otherwise, you will start rambling, and the committee will not understand what you are trying to communicate to them. Don't try to *wing it* with these types of questions.

As mentioned above, behavioral questions can be a setup for you to give too much information. Don't become flattered by the interviewer's interest, or you're going to give way too much information and stray away from the actual question. *For example, It's interesting that you asked how I handle stress. I am thinking about learning a meditation technique, Transcendental Meditation (TM), to help me relax daily and get more in touch with my feelings.*

Uh-oh!

That's why I'm here to help you not look like a phony. First, I will provide a list of common traditional and behavioral questions. Then, I will help you craft some model answers and get you thinking about tailoring your response using your own experiences and frameworks.

When I help applicants prepare for an upcoming interview via my mock interview coaching service, I've come to realize how many applicants are *winging it* out there. However, studies show that those who do mock interviews before the actual interview outperform applicants who don't do a trial run, hands down.

I'm also going to present you with some absolute *no-no's* to avoid. Finally, I'll give some outlines and structure in which you can fit *your* specific information and come off like a professional interviewee, no matter what kind of question they throw at you. I'll provide you with clues about what the interviewer is getting at with her question and how to navigate the dark waters successfully. I'll also give you guidance on what *not* to do.

Keep in mind this mantra; *it's not about you; it's about them,* when preparing your answers to interview questions. If you don't learn anything else from this chapter, this mantra will help you quite a bit. As I mentioned, I will give you special training in being prepared for interview questions, but I'll also provide you with everything else you need to succeed at your PA school interview. Your competition won't stand a chance!

As you'll see in the answers I provide for you, I have underlined the qualities that the answer requires. You should now be familiar with what the qualities are and their importance in the tailoring process. The qualities are underlined.

Also, don't forget about the multipliers: the extra bits of information that will supercharge your answers. I highlight them in bold.

I will also provide a list of *Dos* and *Don'ts* at the end of each answer.

Before starting this section, I want to clarify that **these answers are a guide, and you should not memorize them.** Instead, use the sample answers as a tool, but you're the one who has to do the work to personalize your responses.

THE TRADITIONAL QUESTIONS

"Tell me about yourself"

Chances are very likely that you will be asked this traditional question at your interview, and trust me, and the committee doesn't want to know that you love to meditate on the beach at sunrise or that you're an avid runner. Instead, what they're asking is, why are you a good fit for our program?

Your answer to this question can significantly influence the outcome of your interview. The interviewer(s) wants to know that you have the necessary qualities to precisely fulfill what they're looking for in their *perfect applicant*. If you've done your homework as mentioned above, you will know precisely the core must-haves to get accepted to this program.

When answering this question, you'll want to weave a story that explains how your experiences and skillsets have led you to the PA profession and this program in particular. Show them that you have the qualities they're seeking.

Here is a good answer that will help guide you and help you build your response.

Example Answer

> *I think the best way to do that would be to tell you about a time when I was faced with a pretty stressful situation while working as an EMT. To keep current on procedures and protocols, our squad held four-hour training sessions on Saturdays. Because our supervisor was trying to squeeze too many topics into one session, we all felt overwhelmed and anxious because we couldn't absorb all of the information in that short period. Everyone expressed concerns, but nobody came up with a solution. Finally, because training is so vital to EMTs, I came up with a solution. I suggested we use our Saturday training sessions to cover one topic at a time. I suggested that we break down the individual issues into one every Saturday over three-month blocks of time. Everyone was thrilled*

> *with this idea, and we were able to provide an enhanced learning capacity and reduce the stress and anxiety in the squad. I bring this story up because it highlights two things I pride myself on: solving problems and thinking outside the box.*

Qualities: problem solver and thinking outside the box

DOS:
- ✓ Focus on the strengths the program seeks.
- ✓ Keep the story brief and to the point.
- ✓ Keep the story focused on work accomplishments.

DON'TS:
- ✗ Don't talk about your love for hiking or your passion for playing tennis.
- ✗ Don't stray.
- ✗ Don't focus on personal situations; keep it focused on work accomplishments.
- ✗ Don't recount any situation that occurred over 10 years ago.
- ✗ Don't talk about educational or work experiences that are not relevant to being a solid PA school applicant.
- ✗ Don't open your answer by giving your name and home.

Another way to answer this question would be to incorporate the following dialogue in your answer:

I have been in the _____ industry/field for the past ___ years. My most recent experience has been _____ _____ in the _____ industry/career field. One reason I particularly enjoy this job, and the challenges that go with it, is the opportunity to connect with people/patients. In my last/current job I formed some significant patient relationships resulting in a deeper understanding of what it takes to be a competent medical provider.

My real strength is my ability to _____. I pride myself on my reputation for _____. When I commit to _____, I make sure _____ _____.

What I am looking for now is a profession that values diversity, _____, and _____, where I can use my qualities and strengths to become a competent physician assistant.

"Why should we select you?"

A classic interview question is; *Why should we select you over the other applicants interviewing today?* What makes you unique? The interviewer(s) will usually tell you how competitive the applicant pool is this year, and there are many qualified applicants. You might feel a little disheartened at this point, but don't let it get to you. If you weren't one of those highly qualified applicants, you wouldn't be there. The committee simply wants you to convince them that you have what it takes to be a good fit for their program.

Your goal at the interview is to claim your seat and show the committee that you are the solution to their problem: finding perfect applicants.

Example Answer

> I am uniquely qualified to attend Stanford's PA program because of your program's mission to have its graduates focus on primary care in California and work in underserved communities. I also know that it is essential at Stanford to increase the enrollment and deployment of under-represented minorities. As you can see from my CASPA application, *I have several years of hands-on medical experience working in underserved communities*. It seems to me that the **Stanford Medical School's Free-Clinics** that offer quality health care to underserved populations is incredible. There are so many PA programs that desire applicants to work in underserved areas, but few of them provide the opportunity to do this on campus. My experience working with underserved populations prepares me to hit the ground running in this program.

Quality: the desire to work in underserved areas
Multiplier: Stanford Medical School's Free Clinics

DOS:
  ✓ Show you understand the mission of the program because you have researched their website.
  ✓ Before going to the interview, your research on the program may show you how you best fit the culture.
  ✓ Show that you have experience working in underserved areas, that you don't just talk the talk; you walk the walk.

DON'TS:
  ✗ Don't mention that you have spoken with the other interviewees that morning; you feel you are the most qualified.

✗ Don't brag.

✗ Don't be afraid to reiterate portions of your CASPA application that show you fit their needs.

✗ Don't bring up working in underserved areas if you have no experience doing so. Instead, focus on a different quality.

"What is your greatest weakness?"

Please do not say that *I am a perfectionist* or any other faux weakness that might turn into strengths. And certainly don't tell them that you're an alcoholic, but you are now in recovery. (If they hand you a rope, don't hang yourself with it.) Nevertheless, the question is serious, and it requires an insightful answer. The committee wants to know what areas you've struggled with and what you've done to overcome these shortcomings. To answer this question appropriately, you will have to do a great deal of self-reflection. We all have weaknesses and turn them into positives that work for us; it shows adaptability and insights into our character—two desirable traits to have as a PA student.

Beware. The committee might look at your flaws that fit a pattern of applicants who may have dropped out of the program in the past.

Example Answer

> I tend to be a great starter and a poor finisher when it comes to writing papers. I've learned a different approach to dealing with this issue. For example, when writing papers in college, I would always leave the most difficult, time-consuming research for last, which led to procrastination and anxiety. Now, I've learned that I do much better when I tackle the problematic research first, while I have the most energy, and leave the less time-consuming research until the end, so I won't feel so burdened to complete the paper. I break the project into smaller goals and set a deadline for achieving each one. I know as a student in this program, there is no time for procrastinating. Students cannot afford to fall behind in classwork. I pride myself on being able to examine problems and come up with strategic solutions.

Qualities: self-aware, problem solver

DOS:

✓ Turn a weakness into a strength.

✓ Spend some time reflecting on a legitimate weakness you've identified and how you overcame it.

✓ Make sure you let them know that your fault never gets in the way of your performance and that you know how to strategically correct problems when they do arise.

DON'TS:

✗ Don't tell the committee that you walk on water and have no weaknesses.

✗ Don't use a cliché, faux weakness and try to turn it into a strength.

✗ Don't hang yourself; now is not the time to talk about your alcoholism, arrest record, or the fact that you are a loner.

"What are your goals as a PA?"

This question can be a trap to see if you plan to work in a primary care setting, working with underserved populations, or if your goals are inconsistent with the program's mission. To make this question easy to answer, I advise that you break the goals down into short-, medium-, and long-term goals.

Example Answer

I have short-, medium-, and long-range goals once I become a PA. My short-term goal is to work clinically in the primary care setting with underserved populations. I wish to build on what I've learned in PA school and solidify a strong foundation in medicine that will help me throughout my entire career. My medium-range goal, say five years from now, is to work in research. I worked on many research projects in college, and I strongly desire to continue as a physician assistant. I notice that City College has done some groundbreaking research in PTSD, Alzheimer's, and developing a new aspirin to fight cancer. I have a particular interest in finding a cure for Alzheimer's disease. My long-term goal is to tie in my clinical background, research experiences and one day teach at a PA program. I would like to give back to the profession by helping to educate and motivate students.

Quality: has specific short-, medium-, and long-term goals, which include research.

Multiplier: the groundbreaking research conducted at City College.

DOS:

✓ Break your goals into short-, medium-, and long-range goals.

✓ The applicant has done his homework in researching the program. Therefore, he incorporates his research background into the answer.

✓ Support your answer with a specific example found in your research that the ADCOM will not expect you to know about, i.e., their *groundbreaking research.*

✓ Consider three acceptable scenarios to provide (for goals as a PA) in your answer: practicing clinical medicine (working directly with patients), doing research, and teaching at a PA program.

DON'TS:

✗ Don't tell the ADCOM that you want to start your career in a specialty, like cardiology. This goal is inconsistent with the program's mission and shows that you are close-minded concerning discovering opportunities in the other disciplines you will find on clinical rotations.

✗ Don't forget to research the program before your interview.

✗ Don't discuss anything specific that you cannot support on your CASPA application. For example, if you have no background in research, don't tell the committee that doing research is one of your goals unless you can provide a strong justification for this decision.

Thirty-Five Traditional Questions

1. Why do you want to become a PA?
2. Why do you want to attend our program?
3. What are your goals as a PA?
4. What do you consider your strengths?
5. How would you describe your personality?
6. What experience do you have that qualifies you to join our program?
7. What do you know about our program?
8. What do you value most in a classmate or coworker?
9. How have you stayed current or informed about the PA profession?
10. If I asked your coworkers or fellow students to say three positive things about you, what would they say?
11. If it comes down to you and one other applicant, why should we select you?

12. If we remember one thing about you, what should that be?
13. Have you applied to other programs? Which ones, and why did you choose them?
14. What is a *dependent* practitioner?
15. Why do you want to change careers (if applicable)?
16. Explain your undergraduate grades.
17. If you had a patient with a language barrier, how would you assist the patient?
18. What makes you mad?
19. Tell us something unique about yourself that's not already included in your application.
20. If you could change one thing about the PA profession as you understand it today, what would you change?
21. What do you like to do outside of school?
22. What area of medicine do you see yourself practicing after graduation?
23. Tell us your thoughts on health care reform.
24. Do you think health care reform will be a positive or a negative for PAs? Why or why not?
25. Should all PA programs be master's-level programs?
26. What is the difference between a PA and a nurse practitioner?
27. Where do PAs fit on the hierarchy ladder with nurses, nurse practitioners, physicians, and technicians?
28. Is it important for PAs to join local, regional, and national associations?
29. What do you think the most challenging part of being a PA is going to be?
30. What does integrity mean to you?
31. What is going to keep you from succeeding in this program?
32. If you could go back or forward in time and do anything either in real life, or fiction, what would you change?
33. Who inspired you the most in life and why?
34. What was the last book you read? What was the plot? Was there a hidden message?
35. Name a time when you were dependent on others.

THE BEHAVIORAL QUESTIONS

Most PA programs now utilize behavioral questions as their preferred way to choose top candidates. They allow the interviewers to determine what specific PA school applicants possess particular skills, knowledge, and experience. For example, the interviewers interpret what you say about yourself and your past behavior to indicate how you will behave in the future.

It is in your best interest to demonstrate through the use of recent, relevant examples that you have done similar jobs with proven success.

While traditional interview questions are more straightforward, like, *How do you handle stress?* The same behavioral question would be, *Tell us about a time when you had to handle a stressful situation and how you dealt with it?* The traditional form of this question is straightforward to answer: I exercise/meditate/practice yoga. However, the behavioral question is much more complex and requires an example of a situation or task.

You can immediately recognize a behavioral question by the wording of the question. Here are some examples of how a typical behavioral question may start:

- *Tell me about a time…*
- *Can you give me an example…?*
- *What was the most significant…?*
- *Describe a time when…*

As soon as the interviewer begins a question in this fashion, you should immediately think of, behavioral question. You will need to provide *an interview story* highlighting the different competencies and skillsets the program seeks. The problem is that although many applicants might have a general idea of how to answer these questions, their answers usually come out way too long and unfocused and don't paint the applicant in the best light.

That's why you need to be aware of the behavioral questions you are likely to ask, create stories, and adapt them to relevant competencies related to a PA's attributes.

Here is a list of common behavioral-based interview question topics:

1. Teamwork Interview Questions

    If the role calls for a team player, give specific examples that demonstrate you are a team player.

2. Leadership Interview Questions

   If people may be reporting to you, or if you've had to take charge of a difficult situation at a job, prepare to answer questions about your ability to lead and motivate others.

3. Handling Conflict Interview Questions

   The PA profession requires interaction with patients and multiple health care providers (or challenging situations with other colleagues). Therefore, the interviewer may ask you for examples of how you handled or defused tricky situations.

4. Problem Solving

   Being a PA requires critical thinking skills, and the ADCOM may want to know about challenging issues/situations that require some innovation or outside-the-box thinking.

5. Biggest Failure Interview Questions

   More and more PA school interviewers are asking failure questions. Whether you like it or not, you need to be prepared to have a good answer.

You may have a little more difficulty answering behavioral questions for many recent college graduates who have not hit the workforce yet. Remember that behavioral questions don't have to be related to health care or a past job. Instead, you may need to connect stories from your education, team sports, or volunteer positions. The key is to relate your answer to the qualities sought in a good PA student or PA. For instance, playing college basketball has nothing to do with medicine, but teamwork is necessary to succeed. You can never mention the quality of teamwork, or collaboration enough in a PA school interview.

Here are six rules for answering behavioral questions:

1. Your answer/example must be specific.
2. Your examples should be concise; don't ramble.
3. Your examples should include the action you took.
4. Your examples must demonstrate your role.
5. Your examples should be relevant to the question asked.
6. Your stories must have results.

Preparing for Behavioral Interviews

PA programs have a defined set of skills and *key competencies* they desire in a strong PA school applicant. These skill sets and competencies could include decision-making and problem solving, leadership, motivation, communication, interpersonal skills, critical thinking skills, the ability to work within a team, compassion, the ability to work autonomously, and influence others. In preparation for your PA school interview, research your answers to the following questions:

1. What are the necessary skills and primary *competencies* programs desire in PA students?
2. What skills are necessary to be a physician assistant or a physician assistant student?
3. What makes a successful PA school applicant?
4. What would make an unsuccessful PA school applicant?
5. What is the most challenging part of being a PA?

The STAR Technique

A great way to answer behavioral questions is to use the STAR technique. STAR is an acronym for the Situation/Task, the Action you took, and the Result (or outcome).

For example, you may need to recall when you had to work under stressful conditions (situation or task). To handle the problem, you had to organize your employees/classmates/coworkers and discuss options to achieve a goal (action). Following the plan you developed, you were able to accomplish the goal on time (result). Using the STAR technique process is a powerful way for you to frame your experiences.

Here are few tips for answering behavioral questions:

✓ Don't ramble and go off on tangents.
✓ Listen, listen, and listen! Remember, we have two ears and one mouth for a reason. If you are unsure about what the question is specifically asking for, ask for clarification. When you respond, be sure to recall your past accomplishments in detail.
✓ Practice your behavioral strategies using real-life examples. The last thing you want to do is attempt to *wing it*. By practicing with real-life examples, you will be able to recall your past experiences and accomplishments with confidence at your interview.

The following information explains the STAR technique in detail:

Situation or Task

Describe the situation you were in or the task you were assigned to accomplish a goal. You must describe a specific event or situation, not a generalized description of what you have done in the past. Be sure to give enough detail for the interviewer to understand the scenario. The situation can be an event from a previous job or a volunteer experience relevant to the question.

Action

Describe the action you took, and be sure to keep the focus on yourself. For example, if you discuss a group project or effort, describe what *you* did—not the team's efforts. Don't tell what you might have done; explain what you did.

Result

What happened as a result of your action? How did the situation/task end? What did you accomplish? What did you learn?

Use examples of your past behavior from internships, classes, school projects, activities, team participation, community service, hobbies, and work experience. In addition, feel free to use examples of notable accomplishments, whether professional or personal, such as scoring a winning touchdown in the championship game, being elected to office in an organization, winning a prize for your artwork, surfing a big wave, or raising money for charity. Finally, wherever possible, quantify your results. Numbers always impress committee members.

Remember that many behavioral questions try to uncover how you responded to adverse situations. You'll need to have examples of negative experiences ready, but try to choose negative experiences that you made the best or—better yet, those that had positive outcomes.

Here's an excellent way to prepare for behavioral-based interview questions:

- Identify six to eight examples from your past experiences where you demonstrated behaviors and skills that PA school ADCOMs seek.
- Half of your examples should be positive, like accomplishments or meeting goals.
- The other half should be situations that may have started negatively, but you turned into a positive achieving the best outcome.

- Vary your examples. If you are a college student, examples from high school may be irrelevant. Instead, try to use examples from the past year.
- Use the STAR technique to answer these questions.

The night before your interview is not the time to prepare for behavioral questions. Instead, it would be best if you started preparing for them long before your interview.

In the interview, listen carefully to each question, identify the question as a behavioral question *(Tell us about a time when...?)*, recall a situation you reviewed before your interview about the question, and immediately think STAR technique.

Tell me/us about a time when you had to overcome obstacles to get a job done?

The interview committee wants to know if you can think for yourself and become a problem solver. So, *tell me about a time...* should clue you in immediately that this is a behavioral question.

Example Answer

While in college, I was involved in a group assignment where four of us had to research the hepatitis C virus and prepare our findings for faculty members and students in the science department. I was assigned to this group late in the process. During my first meeting with the group, I quickly realized that although a large chunk of the research they gathered was very thorough, it was not helpful for a presentation. The information was way too technical and not conducive to a PowerPoint presentation for those with no prior knowledge about hepatitis C. Rather than telling the group to start from scratch; I restructured the complex information into a more straightforward format. Everyone agreed with the changes, and we incorporated the data into an effective PowerPoint presentation. We all received an award for our presentation. I take great pride in coming up with simple, practical solutions to seemingly impossible problems.

Quality: problem solver

DOS:

✓ Take a moment to brag a bit. But, although now is the time to show off your problem-solving skills, don't go overboard.

✓ The applicant took what could have been a disastrous research project and turned it into an award-winning presentation. Rather than starting over from scratch, she looked at the data already collected and revised it into a much simpler format that the audience would be able to digest and understand.

✓ This answer lets the interviewer know that she can think outside the box and be a creative problem solver.

DON'TS:

✗ Don't tell a story where you solved all of the world's problems.

✗ Don't over exaggerate your accomplishment.

✗ Don't take credit for something you didn't do.

Tell me about a time when you had to handle a stressful situation?

Stressful situation questions are highly pervasive, and you must have two or three situations prepared. The interviewer is looking for a specific example of a stressful situation you've had to face and how you resolved it. He may also want to see what you consider stressful.

Example Answer

> *I started a new job as a medical assistant in a family practice. After working there for a week, the medical providers complained about the rooms not being stocked appropriately with supplies. A provider would come out in the middle of an office visit and become angry that there were no paper towels, no band-aids, no gauze, etcetera. We all felt like we were walking on eggshells.*
>
> *The office manager held a meeting and came down pretty heavy on all of us. I felt my job might be in jeopardy, and I had only been there for a week.*
>
> *I also had a lot of experience as a medical assistant, and I suggested that the MAs discuss the problem. Then, I proposed that we develop a checklist and place it outside the door of every treatment room. Then, every morning we would all be responsible for completing the inventory and stock the rooms appropriately.*
>
> *This system worked, and the providers were very appreciative. In addition, the office manager complimented me for coming up with the solution and alleviating a constant stress source in the clinic.*

Qualities: ability to handle stress, problem solver, leadership

DOS:

✓ Use a specific, real-life example of a stressful situation.

✓ State the problem.

✓ Describe precisely what you did to solve the problem.

✓ Make yourself the hero without going overboard.

DON'TS:

✗ Don't ramble, keep it brief and related to the problem.

✗ Don't forget to make yourself the hero.

✗ Don't exaggerate.

Tell me about a time when someone in your team didn't do his job and how you resolved the problem?

Being in a health care team requires that everyone in that team works collaboratively. If one employee has difficulty doing her part, it can throw off the entire team and ultimately affect patient care. ADCOMs feel that they are the gatekeepers for the PA profession, as well as their program. Therefore, the committee wants to know that the applicants they select have leadership qualities, which means dealing with situations as they arrive.

Example Answer

At my last position as a supervisor, I managed several other employees, one of whom seemed always to be a step behind the rest of the team and consistently missed deadlines. I took him aside and talked with him. Through our discussion, I discovered that he received a promotion from another department, and the company never gave him the necessary training for his new position. He was terrified to ask for help out of concern that he would lose his job if it became known that he lacked this training. Instead, he had been struggling and essentially learning on his own.

Rather than having him fired, I realized what he needed was a little help. So we worked out a schedule where we could meet up, and I could mentor him. As a result, I retained a valuable employee by working together and helping him go over the materials and learn his job. So now, rather than slowing down the team, he has become an integral member.

Quality: problem-solver, mentorship, leadership

DOS:

✓ Taking responsibility for your team members and ensuring they're all working together is a sign of a good leader.

✓ Motivate with praise, not with intimidation.

✓ Show that you have an open mind and that you can problem solve.

DON'TS:

✗ Don't brag about deceitful techniques you have employed in the past.

✗ Don't be condescending.

Tell me about a time when your communication skills made a difference?

Being an effective communicator is a necessary trait to have if you are a health care provider. PAs communicate with patients every day, sometimes to explain treatment regimens or a diagnosis, and sometimes to persuade patients about why it's essential to lose weight, control their high blood pressure, or manage their diabetes. Effective communicators make better providers.

Example Answer

> *One project I worked on in college involved developing a program dealing with cultural similarities in everyday life. The challenge was to communicate with my team members and get them to be as excited about their roles in the project as I was about my role. First, I met with them individually, drawing out any specific interests relative to the project. Then, I used the information from these individual sessions to assign responsibility to coincide with that interest, allowing me to bring about the best results through a team effort. The feedback from the team was positive. Everyone felt that they made a positive contribution in their unique way. It was worth the extra effort I made to listen to each individual and motivate them to use their strengths to develop the curriculum.*

Qualities: communication, motivator

DOS:
- ✓ Communicating with a team to discuss each individual's strengths is vital to get the most out of their efforts.
- ✓ Show the committee that you can motivate and persuade people.

DON'T:
- ✗ Don't talk about being aggressive.
- ✗ Don't be authoritative, be collaborative.

Twenty-Five Behavioral Questions

1. Tell us about a time when you had to handle a stressful situation?
2. Your application states that you're a hard worker. Give us an example of a time when you worked hard?
3. Describe an interaction you've had with a patient who made an impact on you?
4. Tell us about a time when your communication skills made a difference?

5. Give us an example of a time when you took the initiative?

6. You mentioned that you're good at selling new ideas to your boss and coworkers in your essay. How do you do that?

7. Have you ever been in a situation, at work or in school, where you felt it was necessary to address an ethical issue? Describe the situation.

8. Tell me about a time when you had a disagreement or confrontation with a boss or coworker?

9. If you and a colleague had a personality clash, what would you do to improve it?

10. Do you think it's important to promote team building in an organization? What steps would you take as a PA student to encourage team building in the class?

11. From your perspective, describe what makes a person likable?

12. Describe a time when you tried your hardest to accomplish something, but you still failed?

13. Talk about a time when you had to work closely with someone whose personality was very different from yours?

14. Describe a time when you struggled to build a relationship with someone important. How did you eventually overcome that?

15. We all make mistakes we wish we could take back. Tell us about a time you wish you'd handled a situation differently with a colleague.

16. Tell us about a time you were under a lot of pressure. What was going on, and how did you get through it?

17. Tell us about the first job you ever had. What did you do to learn the ropes?

18. Describe the most difficult ethical situation you've had to overcome?

19. Describe a long-term project that you managed. How did you keep everything moving along on time?

20. Tell us about a time you set a goal for yourself. How did you go about ensuring that you would meet your objective?

21. Give us an example of a time you managed numerous responsibilities. How did you handle that?

22. Give us an example of when you had to explain something fairly complex to a frustrated client/patient/customer. How did you handle this delicate situation?

23. Tell us about your proudest professional accomplishment.
24. Tell us about a time you were dissatisfied with your work. What did you do to make it better?
25. Tell us about a time when you worked under close supervision or extremely loose supervision. How did you handle that?

ETHICAL INTERVIEW QUESTIONS

Having high ethical standards is a must for anyone who works in the health care profession. As PAs, we face ethical challenges every day. We cannot afford to make decisions based on emotion; instead, we have to make decisions based on what is right.

You will be asked ethical questions during your interview. You will be given hypothetical scenarios to evaluate, and you will be expected to choose an answer, along with your justification for your choice.

You cannot study for ethical questions, and you are not expected to know what it's like to be a PA. However, I will present a few scenarios here to give you an idea of what to expect at your interview. There are also many more ethical scenarios, with answers, presented in my book, *How to Ace the Physician Assistant School Interview.*

Sample Ethical Questions

Do you believe all individuals have a right to health care in this country?

Example Answer

> I believe that all people in this country should have access to health care. Therefore, my job as a medical provider would be to provide the highest quality health care for any patient that presents to me for treatment, regardless of her ability to pay.
>
> As far as patients having a *right* to health care, I believe that is a political decision made by legislators and not medical providers.

Qualities: reasoning, nonjudgmental

DOS:

✓ Think the situation through, and realize the limitations of the health care provider.

✓ Mention that health care providers should treat all patients who present to them for care.

DON'TS:

✗ Don't get into a political discussion.

✗ Don't be authoritative, be collaborative.

Tell me about a time when you had to handle an ethical dilemma?

Example Answer

> I saw one of my classmates using a *cheat sheet* to answer the questions during a biochemistry examination.
>
> I always think it is best to confront a person directly if I am concerned about any discrepancy. I approached my classmate after class and said to him; *I feel like you may have been cheating during this exam. Am I correct?* He admitted to me that he was cheating and told me that he had a lapse in judgment. He confided in me that he had difficulty understanding the material and was afraid to ask for help. I realized that I had two options: report him to the professor or help him study for future exams if he needed the help.
>
> I decided to offer him help with the material, and he was very appreciative. I also advised him that if I caught him cheating again, I would have no choice but to report him to the professor.
>
> As it turned out, he accepted my help and did very well for the rest of the semester.
>
> I am the type of person who believes that everyone has lapses of judgment at one time or another, and I believe in giving second chances when appropriate.

Qualities: compassion, being a *natural* person

DOS:

✓ Confront the student before going to the professor.

✓ Be real.

✓ Act with integrity and honesty.

DON'TS:

✗ Compromise your ethics.

✗ Ignore the situation.

✗ Don't accuse the student.

✗ Don't tell the committee what you think they want to hear.

What would you do if you knew your supervising physician was committing Medicare fraud by overbilling for his services?

Example Answer

> I would first ask to speak to my supervising physician in private. I would tell him that I feel he is overbilling Medicare patients and that I am very uncomfortable participating in a practice that uses unethical billing practices. I would advise the physician that ethics is essential to me. If he continued to bill Medicare inappropriately, I would leave the practice and consider reporting his actions to Medicare.

Qualities: integrity, honesty

DOS:

✓ Be true to yourself.

✓ Confront your supervisor first before taking any other actions.

✓ Advise your supervisor of the consequences of his actions and what action you will take if he does not change his unethical practices.

DON'TS:

✗ Don't be afraid to confront anyone acting unethically.

✗ Don't put yourself at risk by ignoring the problem.

✗ Don't be aggressive when speaking about the dilemma.

Fifteen Ethical Questions

1. What do you believe compromises the ethical workplace?
2. Have you worked for a company with a code of conduct and did you have positive or negative experiences there?
3. Have you taken a course or had any training in medical ethics?
4. How does being an ethical individual differ from being an ethical corporation?
5. Would you ever lie for us?
6. Tell us about a time that you were challenged ethically.
7. When you've had ethical issues arise at work, whom did you consult?

8. I see you've worked with people from different cultures. What ethics and values did you find you had in common, and where did you differ?

9. Do you believe that all individuals have a right to health care in this country?

10. What would you do if you witnessed a classmate cheating on a test?

11. What would you do if your supervising physician asked you to write an order for a medication you thought might harm your patient? What would you do?

12. What if a nurse refused to carry out one of your orders?

13. What would you do if you ordered a medication for a patient in the hospital, and you realized you prescribed the wrong medication.

14. What would you do if you walked on the floor one day, and one of the nurses tells you that she saw your friend and colleague of 10 years take controlled medications out of the narcotics locker and put them in his pocket?

15. What would you do if you noticed your supervising physician billing at a higher level for those patients on Medicaid. When you confront him about it, he tells you Medicaid does not reimburse well; he needs to bill at the higher level to make up for lost revenue.

SITUATIONAL INTERVIEW QUESTIONS

Responses to situational questions can make or break an interview. An interviewer uses situational interviewing techniques to elicit specific examples of an applicant's ability to perform under stress, work as a team player, and communicate with colleagues. Additionally, the interviewer will want to know how well you understand the role of a PA.

A coworker tells you in confidence that she plans to call in sick while taking a week's vacation. What would you do and why?

Example Answer

I would tell this coworker that being dishonest to her boss and coworkers is not wise, and being untruthful in her job is wrong. I would explain how we all want more vacation time, but we have to earn it—and that taking this extra time hurts everyone in the department because the person's absence will affect productivity.

Qualities: assertiveness, team player

DOS:

✓ Be assertive, not aggressive.

✓ Point out the situation from a team perspective.

DON'TS:

✗ Don't ignore the situation.

✗ Don't be condescending.

What would you do if the work of a subordinate or team member was not up to expectations?

Example Answer

Luckily, I have quite a bit of previous team experience and have faced this situation a few times in the past—so let me tell you how I've learned to handle the issue. The essential first step in dealing with an underperforming subordinate or team member is honest communication—talking with the person can lead to some surprising discoveries, such as the person not understanding the assigned tasks or being overwhelmed with the assignment. Once I discovered the problem, I could then forge a solution that usually solved the problem and allowed the work to move forward. Unfortunately, in situations like this, the problem is some combination of miscommunications and unrealistic expectations.

Qualities: team player, communicator, problem solver, experienced

DOS:

✓ Communicate directly with the employee.

✓ Be honest.

✓ Consider the problem from both sides.

DON'TS:

✗ Don't go directly to the supervisor without talking to the employee first.

✗ Don't assume your subordinate is purposely underperforming.

How would you deal with a colleague at work with whom you seem to be unable to build a successful working relationship?

Example Answer

> This situation would certainly be unique to me. Ever since I can remember, I've had a knack for finding something in everyone that becomes common ground for a friendship and a good working relationship. Indeed, there are all types of people, some less motivated to work in teams or unhappy in their jobs, but we're all people when you strip away titles and such—and it's at that base level in which I find a connection which results in some degree of rapport—even when few others can do so. For example, in my senior year of college, I was placed on a team with one member that the rest of the team disliked. The team member was an outcast, but I knew we needed this total commitment to make this project work. Even though I was not the team leader, I took it upon myself to forge a connection—and discovered we had a mutual passion for horses. We did not become best friends, but I built enough rapport to connect and engage him as a critical team member through our common interests. There is always something that bonds us all together—it's just more challenging to find with some people than with others.

Qualities: cooperative, leadership, team-oriented, communication skills

DOS:
- ✓ Try to find common ground with the person.
- ✓ Have a positive attitude.
- ✓ Be cooperative.
- ✓ Take the high ground.

DON'TS:
- ✗ Don't ignore the situation.
- ✗ Don't get resentment toward your colleague.
- ✗ Don't forget the goal is teamwork.

Fifteen Sample Situational Questions

1. In health care, we deal with all types of patients and coworkers. Explain how you have dealt with a difficult person at work. How did you handle it? What were the results?

2. What would you do if you ordered a medication for a patient, but the nurse refused to carry it out?

3. What would you do if you worked in the emergency room and wanted to admit a very sick 9-year-old, but the attending physician wanted to send her home?

4. What is the biggest challenge you've faced, and how did you solve it?

5. Describe a time when you had to defend an unpopular decision you made.

6. Describe a recent situation where you dealt with an upset coworker or customer.

7. Tell us about your most challenging boss and how you could deal with them.

8. What would you do if you were working on an important project and suddenly the priorities were changed?

9. Please describe a time when your boss or other coworkers criticized your work.

10. Share with us a time you went the extra mile to resolve a problem or accomplish something.

11. Team members you've been assigned to lead during a new project object to your vision and ideas for implementation. What precisely would you do to address their objections?

12. You're responsible for an important project near completion but receive another vital task to complete. How do you multitask and prioritize?

13. When a subordinate performs below average, what specific steps do you take to correct the problem?

14. You're responsible for ensuring a large amount of work is to be finished before a school project is due. A classmate decides to use sick time to take an entire week off from school. What would you do to address the problem?

15. What would you do if you knew your supervising physician was wrong about a critical work-related issue?

ILLEGAL INTERVIEW QUESTIONS

Similar to writing good test questions, selecting appropriate interview questions is a skill. Many PA school ADCOM members are not professional interviewers and may not even know the rules about illegal interview questions. PA school interview questions should be directed at your qualifications to become a PA and not about your personal information.

When dealing with illegal interview questions, ask yourself: "Do I want to be right, or do I want to be effective?" In other words, if you are asked a question that you know is illegal to ask, you may not want to say, *Hey, that's an illegal question.* Instead, I suggest you assume the interviewer is asking the illegal question out of ignorance and not trip you up.

For this chapter, we'll assume the interviewer is ignorant of the rules about asking illegal questions. So I'll show you how to answer the (underlying) question without exposing any personal information.

What questions are illegal?

- Questions about marital status/family status
- Questions about age
- Personal questions
- Questions about disabilities
- Questions about your arrest record
- Questions about military service
- Questions about politics/affiliations
- Questions about race, color, or religion

Here are some examples of typical illegal questions and answers.

Do you have any children?

[The interviewer may ask you this question to determine in his mind *(fortune-telling)* if you will need to take time off from school or rotations to stay home with your children.]

Example Answer

> There is absolutely no reason I will not show up for a class or clinical rotations every day.

Notice the applicant recognizes this as an illegal question and answers the real question being asked, *Are you going to be missing a lot of time because you don't have daycare?*

How old are you?

(This question probably has more to do with maturity than chronological age.)

> I've accomplished all of the academic prerequisites and health care experience requirements to qualify for this program. I know what it takes to become a good physician assistant, and I am ready to embrace the challenges of PA school.

How much do you weigh?

(This is a rude and illegal question. The interviewer may be thinking you cannot handle the job if you are overweight or obese. The interviewer may also be highly judgmental.)

> Weight has never been an issue for me. I've never had a problem performing any of my job duties.

I see you're not moving your left arm. Did you hurt yourself?

(This is a *fishing* question to see if you have a disability that would interfere with your duties as a PA.)

> I'm fine, thank you.

You have an interesting accent; what is your native country?

(Inquiries about a person's citizenship or country of birth is unlawful and imply discrimination based on national origin.)

> That's an interesting question. Is this information pertinent to my application?

Have you ever been arrested?

(Upon completing PA school, you will have to undergo a background check to see if you qualify for a medical license. If you have any felonies or drug convictions, you will be disqualified. You may want to check this out for yourself before applying to PA school. However, if you have been arrested for minor offenses but not convicted, you don't have to divulge that information. If you have a current arrest, the ADCOM can ask you about that and consider it when deciding your candidacy.)

> No, I've never been convicted of a criminal offense.

Are you a Republican or a Democrat?

(This is a loaded question. Never talk about politics at an interview unless you want to sabotage your chances of being accepted.)

| It's my policy never to discuss politics with anyone. |

What is your religion?

(All religious questions are illegal. However, interviewers may ask about your religious background to see if you will have any conflict working Saturdays or Sundays.)

| My religious preference is very personal. |

Twenty Sample Illegal Questions

1. Are you Caucasian/African American/Hispanic?
2. Do you attend church/synagogue/mosque?
3. Are you married?
4. Are you planning to have children?
5. Are you pregnant?
6. Who is going to watch your children when you are in school?
7. When were you born?
8. When is your birthday?
9. How tall are you?
10. What is your sexual orientation?
11. What medications do you take?
12. Do you have any mental health issues?
13. Do you have heart disease?
14. Have you ever been treated for alcoholism or drug addiction?
15. Do you have an eating disorder?
16. Will you need us to make any accommodations for you to complete the program?
17. Where were you born?
18. Are you a citizen?

19. Your last name sounds Italian, is it?
20. Who did you vote for in the last election?

HYPOTHETICAL QUESTIONS: IF YOU WERE AN ANIMAL/COLOR/FRUIT/TREE, WHAT WOULD IT BE?

It is becoming increasingly common for interviewers to ask unusual questions during interviews rather than sticking to the tried and true. Asking hypothetical questions could be for several reasons: they want to see if you can think on your feet, think creatively, say something illuminating about yourself, and possibly demonstrate a sense of humor.

The following hypothetical questions may seem a bit odd or even a bit ridiculous. You may be asking yourself:

- "What difference does it make what color I would be?"
- "Is this a psychiatric interview or an interview for PA school?"
- "If I say an apple versus an orange, will that answer affect my score?"

How ridiculous, right? Well, you may think these hypothetical questions are foolish. Still, the matter is that programs frequently ask the following hypothetical questions, and the perfect applicant knows how to provide an intelligent answer.

Let's look at some of the most common hypothetical questions and answers.

If you were an animal, what would it be, and why?

> If I were an animal, I would be an eagle. An eagle is a bird that can soar ten thousand feet above the ground and see for three square miles. Yet, at the same time, an eagle can also see the tiniest mouse crawling on the bottom of a desert floor.

The implication is that you can see the *big picture* while also focusing on the minor details.

If you were a color, what would it be, and why?

> If I were a color, I would be charcoal gray. Charcoal gray is a unique color that represents maturity, leadership, and it blends well with any other color.

By choosing charcoal gray as your color, you tell the committee that you are an individual, not a carbon-copy applicant. You are also saying that you are mature and that you're a team player.

Are you starting to see the point? You should choose your answers to coincide with some of the qualities of the perfect applicant.

Let's try another.

If you were a fruit, what would it be?

> I would be a banana. A banana has substance and blends well in a fruit salad.

You tell the committee that you are a strong applicant and that you would be a good classmate (team player).

If you were a tree, what would it be?

> If I were a tree, I would be a palm tree. A palm tree can sway to the ground without breaking in a severe storm, yet it always bounces right back up once the storm is over.

The qualities are flexibility and resilience.

There are no right or wrong answers to hypothetical questions. Your job is to think on your feet and come up with a solution. The answer should include your qualities, and the qualities the ADCOM is looking for in the perfect applicant.

SUMMARY

We covered a lot of ground in this chapter. I hope you now appreciate how much *work* it takes to become the perfect applicant. You learned about the tailoring method and how to find the qualities each program looks for in future students. You also learned about using multipliers to supercharge your answers. You will blow away the competition by infusing qualities and multipliers into the answers you provide at the PA school interview.

But not so fast! Effectively building trust and credibility with the ADCOM involves more than just providing great answers to the interview questions. Answering the questions is only the *verbal* component of your message, and the spoken message has three parts: verbal, vocal, and visual. And believe it or not, the visual and vocal components can weigh much more than the verbal component. So if you are a bit confused, take a look at the next chapter to see exactly what I mean.

[CHAPTER 8]

The Interview (Part Two)

THE MULTIPLE MINI-INTERVIEW (MMI)

In the previous chapter, we've covered almost every possible question you may have to answer at your physician assistant (PA) school interview. However, some programs utilize the MMI (multiple mini-interview). Chances are you've never even heard of the MMI-style interview, let alone participated in one. After an MMI interview, I've spoken with many applicants who feel the MMI is more complicated than traditional interviews. Most of these applicants also admit they did not prepare for the MMI format and naturally didn't do very well. In this chapter, I'm going to cover:

- What is the MMI interview?
- How do I approach the MMI?
- How do I answer MMI questions?
- Review of key points.

There are an infinite number of prompts that you may be asked/given at an MMI interview. Therefore, this chapter will not contain multiple questions with sample answers. Instead, I will cover the four points above and use one single prompt as an example of approaching and answering MMI questions.

What Is the MMI?

The MMI format is the newest type of interview utilized by PA programs. PA programs feel the MMI format is a better indicator of academic and clinical performance. In addition, the MMI better assesses the candidate's nonacademic qualities and the ability to think on her feet.

History of the MMI

In 2004, the Michael DeGroote School of Medicine at McMaster University (Canada) began developing the MMI format to address two widely recognized problems: (1) Traditional interview formats do not accurately predict performance in medical school. (2) The most common patient complaints relate to noncognitive skills, such as interpersonal skills, professionalism, and ethical/moral judgment. McMaster reported that using the MMI format increases the reliability of the interview in assessing an applicant's suitability for the practice of medicine.

Format of the MMI

During an MMI, the interviewee moves from station to station during a designated time period throughout the day. The stations are simply interviewing rooms lined up in a hallway or a circular fashion. Once the applicant completes station one, she moves on to station two. The applicant keeps progressing until she has completed all the designated stations. The number of stations will vary from program to program. Some interviews are occasionally split, with half of the interviews in the MMI format and half in a *traditional* format. Typically, you can expect a full MMI interview to last approximately 2 hours, with breaks.

There are typically six to eight stations during an MMI interview. The interviewee is given anywhere from 6 to 10 minutes to complete a station. Upon arrival at a station, you will find a notecard or piece of paper on the door, with a written prompt on it. The prompt may consist of:

- A scenario that you must discuss when you enter the room.
- A task you must complete inside the room.
- A role-playing scenario.
- A scenario involving a current PA student or administrator.

You will have 2 minutes outside the room to read the prompt and begin to formulate your response. You may be able to take notes, but it is not guaranteed. You should find out *before* your interview if you are

Figure 8.1. Sequence of events during an MMI station

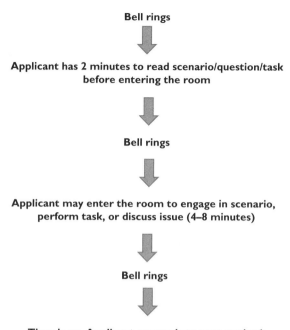

Bell rings

Applicant has 2 minutes to read scenario/question/task
before entering the room

Bell rings

Applicant may enter the room to engage in scenario,
perform task, or discuss issue (4–8 minutes)

Bell rings

Time is up. Applicant proceeds to next station*

*The process continues until the applicant completes all stations.

allowed to take notes or not. After the 2-minute time frame is up, a bell will sound, notifying you that it is time to enter the interview room to discuss the prompt with the interviewer. Once inside the room, you will have from 4 to 8 minutes (depending on the length of the station) to complete your response. Let's review the sequence of events during an MMI station (Figure 8.1).

TIP: Be sure to wear a watch when you come for your interview. Most likely, there will not be a clock in the hallway or inside the room. The last thing you want to have happened is having the bell go off inside the room when you are trying to wrap up an answer. When the bell rings, you stop!

The Goal of the MMI

The goal of the MMI is to assess your nonacademic qualities and your ability to think and react quickly.

Why MMI *over* Traditional Interview?

To assess nonacademic qualities. The interviewer assesses these qualities at each station.

See Table 8.1 for a list of qualities most assessed by admissions committees.

There Are No Right or Wrong Answers

Applicants are all graded on a spectrum, which allows for a better comparison of candidates.

MMIs Minimize Examiner Bias

- Multiple independent assessors and stations
- Flexibility in scenarios
- Allows for recovery in a disastrous station

Why Is the MMI Important?

Most applicants selected for a PA school interview have high GPAs, excellent test scores, and much medical experience. The MMI is a way to distinguish yourself from the other highly qualified applicants. Once you reach your interview, it can be the single most crucial aspect of your application.

How to Approach the MMI

At each station, be prepared to respond to one of the following prompts. Of course, you will need to know what to say and how to say it. Here are a few common prompts that you may receive:

- Ethical dilemma
- Knowledge of PA profession/health care
- Role-playing scenarios
- Task station

Example of an Ethical Dilemma

An attending physician is in the habit of introducing PAs rotating with him as *doctors*. Discuss the ethical issues raised by this practice.

Table 8.1. Personal Characteristics Assessed During the Admissions Interview

Characteristics	Percentage
Motivation for a medical career	98%
Compassion and empathy	96%
Personal maturity	92%
Oral communication	91%
Service orientation	89%
Professionalism	88%
Altruism (selflessness)	83%
Integrity	82%
Leadership	80%
Intellectual curiosity	76%
Teamwork	74%
Cultural competence	72%
Reliability and dependability	70%
Self-discipline	70%
Critical thinking	69%
Adaptability	67%
Verbal reasoning	66%
Work habits	66%
Persistence	65%
Resilience	65%
Logical reasoning	56%

Source: Adapted from the Association of American Medical Colleges (AAMC), www.aamc.org

Example of Knowledge of the PA Profession

Talk about Full Practice Authority and Responsibility (FPAR) as it relates to the PA profession. Are you for FPAR or against it? How do you think it will change the PA profession?

NOTE: If you do not know what FPAR means to the PA profession, Google *AAPA Task Force and FPAR* for a summary.

Example of Role-Playing Scenario

You work in a family practice clinic. The next patient on your schedule is Mr. Jones. You must inform Mr. Jones that his recent CT scan shows that he has cancer in his pancreas with metastases to other parts of his body. How would you break the sad news?

Example of a Task Station

You walk into the station and find a pair of sterile gloves on the table and instructions for putting them on. A PA student is sitting across the table from you. The student also has a pair of sterile gloves in front of him. Your task is to teach/explain to the other applicant how to put the gloves on sterilely.

Scoring Your Performance

The interviewer(s) will observe and score your performance. All interviewees that day experience the same questions, scenarios, and tasks for consistency. Keep in mind that in an MMI interview, you can see any number of prompts. Here are some other examples of MMI prompts you may encounter.

- Discuss your past experiences with PAs.
- Why are you a good fit for the PA profession? Would you please discuss your qualifications and experiences?
- What are your biggest strengths and weaknesses?
- Write a letter to a professor about a bad grade (D+) you received on your final paper of the semester. The professor's comments state that your grammar was an issue, and the topic's analysis was superficial.

- Anatomy station: Write out blood flow through the systemic circulation, starting with the inferior vena cava.
- Anatomy station: There may be a model of the knee on the table. Label as many structures as you can.
- Role playing: You are a phlebotomist in a hospital. Treat this room as if you are with a patient with whom you struggled to get blood. You must retake more blood because you drew the original sample into the wrong colored tube. How would you deal with this situation? Also, describe the difference between sympathy and empathy.
- If one student in your group project cheated, should all the students in the group fail?
- You must choose a punishment and level of discipline for a professional infraction. For the type of punishment, the choices include:

  1. Verbal warning
  2. Written warning
  3. Probation
  4. Dismissal

  For the *level* of punishment, your choices are:

  1. Mild
  2. Moderate
  3. Severe
  4. None

  The infractions include:

  1. Dishonesty
  2. Informally addressing a superior
  3. Plagiarism

As you can see from the examples above, you may have to address several prompts at your MMI interview. One issue you may encounter is fatigue from the volume of prompts you will discuss on interview day. I strongly recommend that you practice MMI scenarios a few weeks before your actual interview. You can start with one per day for a week, then increase the number of prompts and answers at your own pace. I also recommend increasing the number of prompts until you can answer six to eight prompts in one sitting. Do not try to memorize answers or practice scenarios; there is too much variation between the programs.

Responding to an MMI Prompt

- What to say
- How to say it

What to Say in Your Response

The Four Pillars of Medical Ethics:

1. **Autonomy** refers to the capacity to think, decide, and act on one's free initiative. The PA profession has always embraced this concept.
2. **Beneficence** (charity, mercy, kindness) involves promoting what is best for the patient given all viable options and complicating factors.
3. **Non-maleficence** (non-harming) refers to the principle of first *do no harm* and could be encompassed under beneficence.
4. **Justice** is the science and art of prioritizing the distribution of limited resources.

Professional Competency Roles

- Professional
- Communicator
- Manager
- Health advocate
- Scholar
- Health care system/training in the field
- Almost all prompts can be related to health care
- Show how you could apply a scenario to health care

Example: How to incorporate the health care system into your response

Health care system: The prompt asks you what you would do if you walked out of your front door one day and found a shoebox with $100,000 in it. There is no note and no identifying information on the box.

At first glance, it's not obvious how you might bring the health care system into this discussion. However, if not done correctly, your answer can seem forced and off-point.

It takes a lot of practice and thinking on your feet to incorporate these points strategically and may not be appropriate for every scenario.

Response

After providing a complete answer to the prompt question, you could add the following:

While the decision-making process in this example is challenging, I would imagine that health care providers are faced with even more significant challenges every day. For example, here, I might have to advise a patient that there are many courses of treatment to consider for his illness, each having pros and cons.

I would approach the conversation regarding treatment options using similar strategies I discussed when deciding what to do with the money.

Connecting a general prompt to health care is a beautiful way to highlight your potential as a PA student and future PA.

It is also a great idea to incorporate some of your past individual experiences when answering the prompt.

Responding well to a hypothetical ethical scenario is excellent, but *demonstrating* that you've had success using these techniques in the real world can make your answer even more potent, and in some cases, more compelling.

Let's build off our example above on deciding what to do with the $100,000 you found on your doorstep. After answering the question, you may want to bring in a personal experience.

Example: How to incorporate a personal experience into your prompt

After graduating college, I joined a church group. One day a single mom joined the group, and it was apparent she was struggling with finances. She had recently lived in a shelter with her three children and struggled to feed and clothe them. So one day, I decided to purchase groceries for her and clothes for the kids. I left the packages on her front step and left. I've always liked doing things for people and not getting caught.

By relating the prompts to your own experiences, you prove to the interviewer that you possess the qualities valuable to a competent medical provider. Learning to incorporate the health care system and personal experiences into the answers to prompts takes a great deal of practice.

How to Say It: Strategies for Dealing with a Prompt

Now that we have discussed what to say when responding to an MMI prompt, let's explore how to say it. Here are four strategies for dealing with a prompt:

1. Know what the prompt is asking. The worst thing you can do is not answer the question. Many applicants I coach do this a lot when I ask them, "Why do you want to become a PA?" They tell me that "I've always been fascinated by science, love helping people, and am a team player." But, they never answer the specific question, "Why do you want to become a PA?" The answers above could be relevant to becoming a paramedic, nurse, physician, or medical assistant.

2. Manage your time. It will take a considerable amount of practice to answer a prompt in 6 or 8 minutes. Again, make sure you wear a watch to the interview. It's natural to become nervous about this process with an infinite number of possible prompts and the MMI's stress. It is also essential to learn how to manage your anxiety. Having a structure in place to answer the prompts will go a long way to calm your nerves.

When you first start practicing answering MMI prompts, you will probably find that you will not be able to fill the time. Then, as you practice a little more, you'll probably find that you have too much to discuss. At this point, you are well practiced at viewing prompts from different perspectives. Now is when you need to learn to focus on the most salient points.

3. Formulate a strategy for answering the prompt. It is imperative to have a plan for breaking down a prompt into its most essential parts. It also gives structure for how to develop and deliver your content promptly.

I find the best strategy for answering a prompt is to:

- First, identify the issues/actors and missing information.
- Consider the problems from multiple perspectives before starting your answer.
- End effectively.

(Later in this chapter, I'll illustrate how to use this strategy by providing examples.)

4. Listen for feedback and follow-up prompts from your interviewer. The interviewer may ask you follow-up questions. Again, this is an excellent opportunity to turn a monologue into a dialogue.

In addition, interviewers may have questions they want to ask at the end of your response or throughout your answer. By doing so, they can test your ability to listen, and it is also an opportunity for you to showcase your ability to adapt to additional information.

Being an effective listener is a quality that you will need to be an effective clinician. You must listen to your patients and not just talk to them.

HOW TO ANSWER MMI QUESTIONS

Let's now look at an MMI prompt and how to answer it using what we've learned so far.

Outside the Room (2–3 minutes)

Example Prompt

The PA profession has long debated whether to change the profession's title from physician assistant to physician associate. Many PAs feel that the word assistant does not accurately reflect PAs' advanced training and abilities, and they think patients may mistake them as medical assistants. If you frequent the PA Forum (physicianassistantforum.com), you will find various comments on this topic. Most favor changing the name to physician associate.

In a small poll posted on *Inside PA Training's* website (mypatraining. com), 507 participants voted on this topic. Here are the results:

- Three hundred and sixty participants (71.01%) voted to change the name to *physician associate.*
- Seventy-nine participants (15.58%) voted not to change the name.
- Sixty participants (13.41%) voted to change the title but not to *physician associate.*

If you had the tie-breaking vote on choosing to keep the name or change the name, how would you vote and why? Would you change the name to physician associate? Would you change the name to something else? Would you keep the name as it is? Who would you consider before making your decision?

Questions to Think About

1. Do you think PAs should vote to change the profession's name to *physician associate?*
2. Should PAs vote to change the name or keep it the same?
3. Should PAs vote to choose a different name for the PA profession?
4. What is your opinion on changing the name?
5. Who would you consult/consider when making this decision?

Set a timer for 2 minutes and prepare your response.

This exercise may seem completely overwhelming at first. Don't worry! This is most likely the first time you've had to answer an MMI prompt, and formulating a response to this answer in 2 minutes is a challenging task. You may be thinking, "How am I going to plan an 8-minute response in 2 or 3 minutes?" The answer is to read on, and practice, practice, practice.

It will make it much easier to plan what you'd like to say inside the room in such a brief time frame with more practice.

Inside the Room (6–8 minutes)

Summarize the Prompt

Always start with a summary of the prompt. You want to make sure that you understand the prompt correctly and that you're on the same page with the interviewer. For example, by asking, "Do I have this right?" At the end of your summary, you'll get the dialogue started with the interviewer.

Example

Let's look at a possibility for a summary statement:

The prompt asks me to discuss my thoughts about considering a name change for the PA profession. The question is whether PAs should change the profession's name to *physician associate,* keep the name as it is, or vote to change the name to something other than *physician associate.* The prompt also asks my opinion about who should be consulted or considered about the name change. Do I have this correct?

Summarizing the prompt is also a terrific way to *break the ice.* It could be very intimidating if you're in the room for 6 to 8 minutes with an interviewer who is silent and unresponsive. More importantly, starting with the prompt's summary and asking, "Do I have this right?" is a great way to know if you may have interpreted the prompt differently than the interviewer.

I now want you to go back to the above prompt and summarize the critical points in 15 seconds. Set a timer and see how well you do.

- Should PAs vote to change the name of the PA profession to physician associate?
- Should PAs keep the name as it is?
- Should PAs vote to choose a different name for the PA profession?
- What is your opinion on changing the name?
- Who should I consult/consider concerning the name change?

Notice how concise the summary is and how it gets right to the point. I bet that was a lot simpler than you thought it would be. When you ask the interviewer, "Do I have this correct?" You start a dialogue, and you can be rest assured you're on the right track.

Once you summarize the prompt, the next step is to employ your strategy for answering the prompt. I recommend a method that you've already used when writing a traditional six-paragraph essay. Start with an opening statement, which would be equivalent to your opening paragraph in a narrative statement.

In this case, the introduction should include identifying the actors/ issues and any missing information. Also, you should determine if there are any ethical considerations. It is a good idea to state this information explicitly, so the interviewer understands your thought process. The introductory paragraph should also include a mini-outline for the rest of your answer. It tells the interviewer what you are going to discuss in the remainder of your response. The last sentence should also contain a transitional *hook,* which takes you to the body of your answer.

Next, use a few paragraphs for the body of your answer. Use a topic sentence and a few sentences to support your topic sentence, and then use a transition sentence to the next paragraph. Next, use three or four sections in the body of your answer. Finally, end with a firm summary/ conclusion.

Explicitly identify the key players involved in the scenario and any participants affected by the players' actions.

Provide the Body of Your Answer

The body of your answer is where we identify:

- Who are the key actors and stakeholders involved in the scenario?
- Is there any missing information or unknown parts of the prompt?
- Are there any questions needing clarification?
- Make assumptions and continue. Here is the same prompt again. Try to find the actors, missing information, and critical issues.

Example

The PA profession has long debated whether to change the profession's name from physician assistant to physician associate. Many PAs feel that the word assistant does not accurately reflect PAs' advanced training and abilities, and they think patients may mistake them as medical assistants. If you frequent the PA Forum (physicianassistantforum.com), you will find various comments on this topic. Most favor changing the name to physician associate. In a small poll posted on Inside PA Training's website (mypatraining.com), 507 participants voted on this topic. Here are the results:

- – Three hundred and sixty participants (71.01%) voted to change the name to physician associate.
- – Seventy-nine participants (15.58%) voted not to change the name.
- – Sixty participants (13.41%) voted to change the title but not to physician associate.

If you had the tie-breaking vote on choosing to keep the name or change the name, how would you vote and why? Would you change the name to physician associate? Would you change the name to something else? Would you keep the name as it is? Who would you consider before making your decision?

The Actors, the Missing Information, and the Issues

- Should PA students, as well as practicing PAs, be allowed to vote on a name change?
- Would a much larger sample of voters yield the same results as the small sample used in the above poll?

- What about PA program faculty? Should they have a vote?
- How would physicians react to the name change?

What About the Public?

- How well would patients accept the name change?
- Would patients become confused by a name change?
- How long would it take to reeducate patients?
- Would a name change improve patient satisfaction?
- Is a name change about ego or clarity of the profession?

What About the Profession Itself?

- The Bureau of Labor Statistics (BLS) projects the PA profession to grow 37% from 2016 to 2026. Would the growth rate increase because of a name change?
- The BLS has consistently ranked the PA profession as one of the top career fields. Would changing the name increase the ranking of the profession?
- Would PA salaries increase due to a name change?
- Would PAs be more respected by other health care providers with a name change?

Logistics of a Name Change

How much money would be needed to change the name of the profession? Changing the name of the job would financially impact:

- The American Academy of Physician Assistants (AAPA)
- Every state chapter of the AAPA
- The National Commission on Certification of Physician Assistants (NCCPA)
- CASPA applications, and the Physician Assistant Education Association (PAEA)

Think about the cost, alone, to change every piece of literature? All this information would change the way you answer this prompt.

I provided a list of examples for illustrative purposes only so that you can see the talking points you may want to use during the body of your answer. The actual MMI only focuses on bringing up missing information that you believe would alter your response rather than a laundry list.

For example, how would physicians react to a name change? The name *physician associate* is not a new concept. Although initially, when the profession began, physicians weren't too fond of that name (and were perhaps threatened), PAs at that time changed the name to *physician assistant*. Would the same situation occur if the name is changed now?

Ask the interviewer, "Can you provide me with any more information about any of these questions I just raised?" In many cases, the interviewer will not provide additional information. If she doesn't, quickly state your assumptions so you can move forward efficiently with your response.

Example

Let's look at the prompt again and consider the issues from multiple perspectives. This information will provide the body of your response.

The PA profession has long debated whether to change the profession's name from physician assistant to physician associate. Many PAs feel that the word assistant does not accurately reflect PAs' advanced training and abilities, and they think patients mistake them as medical assistants. If you frequent the PA Forum (physicianassistantforum.com), you will find various comments on this topic. Most favor changing the name to physician associate. In a small poll posted on Inside PA Training's website (mypatraining.com), 507 participants voted on this topic. Here are the results:

- Three hundred sixty participants (71.01%) voted to change the name to physician associate.
- Seventy-nine participants (15.58%) voted not to change the name.
- Sixty participants (13.41%) voted to change the title but not to physician associate.

If you had the tie-breaking vote on choosing to keep the name or change the name, how would you vote and why? Would you change the name to *physician associate*? Would you change the name to something else? Would you keep the name as it is? Who would you consider before making your decision?

Example From Multiple Perspectives

The Actors, the Missing Information, and the Issues

Vote to change the name of the profession.
A vote on a name change is a national issue and will include as many PAs as possible. However, the sample poll mentioned in the prompt only consists of 507 voters, which is not large enough to rely upon, and certainly doesn't capture the opinions of the entire PA profession. Using a larger voting pool, such as PA students, PA Faculty, and the AAPA, may yield a different result .

I would also be very interested as to why the voters would choose to change the name. Is it an ego issue, or is the reason related to more principal issues?

Vote to change the name to something different.
I think there should also be a discussion among PAs about other options for a name change. For example, some PAs have suggested simply using *PA* as the name of the profession. However, I feel that it is still essential to poll PAs about changing the title, and just as important would be to consider the reason for the name change. For example, the poll should include the *reason* why the voter would change the name.

Consider the public.
The PA profession enjoys high patient satisfaction ratings, right up there with nurse practitioners and physicians. PAs enjoy higher-than-average salaries than their college graduate colleagues, and the BLS continues to rank the future of the PA profession as very promising. PAs have also done a remarkable job of educating patients over many years about their role and how they fit into the health care system. Would a name change set the profession back by causing more confusion with patients? Would PAs have to spend years re-educating patients? On the other hand, would a name change provide the profession with even higher satisfaction ratings? I believe having patient focus groups might give more clarity to these questions.

What would be the benefit?

- Higher salaries?
- An even better satisfaction rating?
- A higher score by BLS?
- Better patient care?

I think there may be more questions than answers.

Consider physicians' response to a name change.
Early in the profession, physicians were responsible for the title change from *physician associate* to *physician assistant*. They felt threatened by the name *physician associate* and thought the name might be confusing to patients. It might be a clever idea to include physicians in the process if a name change occurs. Taking this step could avoid the same dilemma in the future if the name is changed.

Consider the logistics of a name change.
Once a name change occurs, the profession will have a financial burden to change the name on every website, administrative agency, and PA program. All the current literature relating to the PA profession would have to be discarded and redone to reflect the new name, whether physician associate or another name. The costs and logistics of doing so would have to justify the name change. There would have to be a thorough investigation on the financial component to weigh the pros and cons of the name change.

My experience.
NOTE: As mentioned previously, it's a good idea to include a personal experience in your answer. Using a personal example shows that you have experience with these issues, and you understand the issues brought up in the prompt and the most effective way of dealing with them.

Concluding Your Response

Hopefully, you feel a little more comfortable now that you have a blueprint for answering MMI questions and showing how the actors and stakeholders are affected. Of course, the next step in the process is the conclusion of your response.

At the end of your response, you'll want to make sure that you end effectively. You've already stated that the prompt is missing some information that could change your answer, and you've noted the relative assumptions that will impact your response. Now arrive at your conclusion that makes sense given the analysis you've already provided:

- Relate the prompt to health care.
- Use a personal example.
- Extend the dialogue.
- Summarize.

A possible conclusion to this prompt could be:

Changing the name of the PA profession from physician assistant to physician associate has been up for debate for several years. The PA profession celebrated 50 years in October 2017. The profession is also consistently ranked as one of the top ten professions by the BLS. One option to consider is, **If it ain't broke, why fix it?**

Changing the name may have a significant impact on the PA profession. I think the AAPA would probably need to set up a task force to consider the implications of changing the name. It will also be important when considering a name change to ask **why** *to change the name? What is the reason for a name change now?*

Additionally, before the name is changed, there would have to be a consensus among PAs. The vote should be open to additional name suggestions for the profession. After a vote, physician associate may not be the choice. Perhaps simply PA would be an appropriate name? After all, many nurse practitioners address themselves as APRNs. Patients are already familiar and comfortable with the name PA, and the word assistant, which seems to be of concern to so many current PAs, would be eliminated.

The profession should also include the public (patients) before making any decisions. Over the past 50 years, PAs have effectively educated the public about the PA profession. As a result, the profession currently enjoys a high satisfaction rating equal to NPs and physicians. PAs should consider whether a name change will confuse patients. Educating the public on a new name could be a considerable challenge. Will a name change upset patients? I hope patients have an active role in the focus groups.

PAs also need to consider that physicians rejected the title physician associate in the early years. Therefore, I believe any focus groups should also include physicians. It would be beneficial to get the physicians' point of view and have a preliminary opinion from physician focus groups on the name change before investing the resources to choose and change the name. I'm happy to get this question/prompt. I have experience working on focus groups while being a Patient Relations Representative in a large city hospital. We often invited patients to participate in the focus groups to see what the hospital was doing right and areas where we could improve. This process was a tremendous learning experience.

In summary, there are much missing information and actors involved, making it difficult for me to give a direct answer. There seem to be more questions than answers. I will favor a name change if FPAR gets granted nationwide. I would vote to change the name to physician associate, but I would also be open to other titles.

To conclude your answer to the prompt, you will need a strong ending. First, provide a clear summary of your talking points. Providing an overview is an excellent way to end our response effectively as it reinforces the most substantial ideas from your response and leaves a positive lasting impression. Take a moment to decide how you would conclude. Next, relate this prompt to yourself and summarize the talking points. The next thing you will want to do after completing your response is to ask follow-up questions. Asking follow-up questions allows you to extend the dialogue with the interviewer. By opening the discussion, you can use the skills you learned from Chapter 9, "Winning Through High Impact Communication," to come across as likable, credible, and trustworthy. Because MMIs tend to be very stressful, do your best to make a positive impression on your interviewer:

- Smile.
- Make eye contact.
- Use open gestures.
- Breathe! Additionally, to keep your anxiety to a minimum, don't forget to use the SHIELD technique (presented in an earlier chapter) before entering the room or at each break. Utilizing this technique will lower your adrenaline levels and keep you out of *fight or flight mode.*

Finally, don't forget that you may also have a role-playing scenario in addition to question-type prompts, or you may have to label the structures on a body part or even teach someone how to perform a specific task.

Follow-Up Questions

Allow time for follow-up questions, as applicable. Remember, it is advantageous to turn a monologue into a dialogue. Answering follow-up questions allows the interviewer to speak and clarify any number of issues you've raised. A follow-up question is also an opportunity for you to show your ability to adapt quickly.

Review Outside the Room

Take the 2 or 3 minutes allowed to read the prompt, reread it, and plan a response based on the skills the prompt is trying to elicit. Develop bullet points to help you structure your answer. Consider the actors, issues, missing information, and multiple perspectives.

Inside the Room

Start by giving a summary of the prompt, and ask, "Do I have this right?" By asking this question, you ensure that you and the interviewer are on the same page. Next, consider the essential parts of the prompt, then analyze and present those parts. These will be the bullet points you developed outside of the room. Next, consider who the actors are and any missing information, and consider the prompt from multiple perspectives. Finally, end effectively by arriving at a conclusion and supporting your argument through personal examples. Then, extend the dialogue by examining follow-up opportunities.

Then, allow time to respond to any of the interviewer's follow-up questions. Remember: In the traditional questions chapters, I stressed the importance of qualities. So, be sure to incorporate as many of your qualities as possible into your answer.

Final thoughts: I hope I have demystified the MMI for you. It is a challenging interview format, and those best prepared will score the highest. Before attending an MMI format interview, try finding out the duration of the stations, both inside and outside the room, the number of stations, the number of rest breaks, the length of the entire interview, and if you will be allowed to take notes and use them inside the room. Don't be afraid to call the program directly to find out this information.

You can also check the program's website, Facebook page, or even go on the PA Forum (physicianassistantforum.com) and check for any information from students or other applicants who may have interviewed at the program. Although most applicants view the MMI interview favorably, a considerable number of applicants have shared with me that their experience was concerning. There are four typical areas of concern my coaching applicants have reported back to me:

1. Lack of control. Many applicants feel that they didn't have enough time to talk about work experience, personal interests, and qualities. They also think that 5 or 6 minutes was not enough time to complete their thoughts fully.

2. Anxiety and nervousness. Some applicants report being so nervous and anxious that they could not think clearly and cohesively communicate their thoughts.

3. Inability to move past inferior performance on a previous station. If an applicant felt she did not do well on the previous station, she could not let go and stay in the moment at subsequent stations.

4. Approach taken by interviewers. Some applicants report being intimidated by the aggressiveness of one or more of the interviewers. Remember, the only way to provide compelling answers to MMI prompts is to practice. The MMI is not an interview where you can *wing it.*

CHAPTER 9

The Interview (Part Three): High-Impact Communication: How to Make an Emotional Connection at your Interview

Now that you've learned the tailoring method to infuse qualities and multipliers into the physician assistant (PA) school interview answers, it's time to look at another essential aspect of the process. In addition to answering questions, the admissions committee (ADCOM) also wants to learn more about you as a person. For instance:

- Are you likable?
- Are you a compassionate person?
- Do you fully understand the role of a PA?
- Are you mature?
- Can you handle stress?
- Can the interviewer(s) visualize you as a colleague?

- Are you overconfident or have a sense of entitlement?
- Are you trustworthy?
- Are you energetic?
- Are you an effective communicator?
- Would the interviewer want you to take care of his mother?

HIGH-IMPACT COMMUNICATION

To claim your seat in next year's class, you will need to develop specific skills and behaviors to enhance your position with the interview committee. The first of these behaviors is charisma or having extraordinary personal power or charm. To some, charisma comes naturally, but more often than not, it must be learned. Charisma results from a series of behaviors through which someone has a powerful and positive impact on others. This is exactly what you want to accomplish at your interview; use charisma to build the bridge to credibility and trust.

As a prior ADCOM member, I've interviewed many applicants who simply could not make that personal connection at the interview. These applicants looked great on paper, or they wouldn't have made it to the interview phase. However, these applicants could not move beyond facts, figures, and jargon to make a connection. In contrast, the applicants who scored highest at the interview knew how to communicate effectively and persuasively, and above all, they were believable. They understood how to project openness, enthusiasm, and energy. The ability to communicate effectively is the single most crucial skill you need to succeed as a PA. I think we've all had an experience with a medical provider who was very dry and impersonal. She may have graduated from Harvard, but if you don't connect with her at a personal level, you may not return for another visit.

Communication is a contact sport. As I mentioned already, looking good on paper will only get you so far. If you cannot make an emotional connection with your audience, you're likely to be rejected. I witnessed this phenomenon over and over again. In contrast, I interviewed many applicants who looked average on paper. Still, they made such an emotional impact at the interview I scored them higher than I had anticipated based on their application alone. Creating an emotional connection with your interviewer(s) is crucial to your success.

CREATING EMOTIONAL IMPACT

It would help if you learned to *sell* yourself to create an emotional impact. You may be thinking, "Sell myself? I'm not a salesperson." Really? Don't you have to sell your ideas to people daily? I know that I have to sell my children why it's essential to do their homework and perform well in school. I sell my patients why it's necessary to take their cholesterol medication or risk getting heart disease. I sell my obese patients why it's important to lose weight if they want to live a long, healthy life. Finally, and most importantly, I have to sell my wife why I want to spend a lot of money on a new toy! We're *all* selling something!

What are you selling? Have you thought about it? I know many of you are uncomfortable with the word "selling." First, however, you will have to sell yourself to the ADCOM at your interview. Second, you will have to give them a good reason why you deserve a seat in the upcoming class among all of the competition. Using the tailoring method introduced in Chapter 7 to answer the interview questions is a good start. But as you'll see, providing exceptional answers to the interview questions is only a tiny piece of the puzzle.

THE SECRET

If you understand that you need to sell yourself to the ADCOM, then make sure you also understand this critical point: *The ADCOM selects candidates based on emotion (likability, credibility, and trust) and justifies that decision with the facts (Grade Point Average [GPA], Graduate Record Examination [GRE] scores, medical experience).* If you understand this simple secret, you will know why you cannot rely on your Centralized Application Service for Physician Assistants (CASPA) application alone at your interview, nor can you rely on the answers you provide to the interview questions. You must make an emotional connection with the committee members to seal the deal.

For example, applicant #1 and applicant #2 come to the interview with the same GPA, GRE scores, medical experience, and volunteer hours. During applicant #1's interview, his answers to the interview questions were perfect. However, he fails to make eye contact; he is not wearing a suit, rarely smiles, and speaks in a monotone voice. Applicant #2 comes in wearing a clean and well-pressed suit; she has a big, genuine smile on her face, looks everyone in the eye when answering the questions, and has excellent intonation and inflection in her voice. She is also spot on with her answers to the interview questions.

After these applicants leave the interview room, the committee does not take out a piece of paper and compare the facts: grades, test scores, answers to interview questions, etc. Instead, they make their decision based on emotion and justify the decision with the facts. When applicant #1 leaves the room, the committee member(s) might say, "I didn't like him, and I'm not crazy about his medical experience." When applicant #2 leaves the room, they might say, "Wow, I like her, and she has excellent medical experience, a great GPA, and GRE scores." Applicant #2 is going to score much higher than applicant #1.

Yes, on paper, both applicants are identical. However, applicant #2 used high-impact communication skills to make that emotional connection and scored higher than applicant #1 with the same credentials. And notice how they justify their decision: "...and she has excellent medical experience, a great GPA, and GRE scores." So remember, they both have identical stats on paper!

In my 3 years on Yale's ADCOM, we made our decisions the same way; "I like her," "I don't like her." Connecting with the emotional center of the interviewer's brain is the key to success!

Three Key Points to Remember

Creating emotional impact is crucial to your success as a PA school applicant. Personal impact is a powerful way to achieve whatever you want in your personal life and career. Consider these three critical points before interviewing:

1. **The spoken word is almost the exact opposite of the written word**

   The written word is a one-dimensional medium for communicating facts and transferring information. However, the spoken word is multidimensional and includes a kaleidoscope of nonverbal cues such as posture, eye contact, energy, volume, intonation, and much more. Therefore, if you want to make an emotional impact and motivate and persuade the ADCOM, you must master the spoken word and learn to make such nonverbal cues work for you rather than against you.

2. **What you say must be believed for it to have an impact**

   If the committee senses that you are less than forthright with even one interview question, you will build a wall of distrust that you probably will not be able to overcome. If they believe you, they'll believe your message.

I once interviewed a woman who applied to Yale's program, and she was in a group interview with myself and two other female ADCOM members. She was a nontraditional applicant, an accomplished, Off-Broadway actress. Unfortunately, she presented us with a very fancy and off-beat résumé (which we didn't ask for, by the way). Located on the bottom right-hand corner of the résumé, below all of her Off-Broadway credits, she wrote, "Special Talents: I can tie a cherry stem into a knot with my tongue." Although this particular talent may be relevant to her role as an actress, it was utterly inappropriate for a PA school application. She had already lost her credibility with my fellow interviewers and me before she stepped foot into the interview room.

One of my colleagues who weren't too pleased with that note on her résumé asked the applicant to comment on her "most memorable patient." The applicant started to cry and talk about her mother's diagnosis of cancer. After the applicant explained that her mother had been in remission for several years, my colleague asked her point-blank, "How do we know you're not acting now?" The silence was awkward. She stopped crying, and she knew the interview was over at that point. She lost her credibility before she even stepped into the room.

A person's gut feeling about whether they like and believe someone is usually based on emotion, not logic. If your voice cracks or your hands are fidgety, or you cannot make solid eye contact, you'll probably lose credibility with your audience.

3. Believability is determined at the subconscious level

Perhaps this is the most vital point to remember. How do we determine whether we believe someone? Can you build believability out of a mountain of facts and figures? No, you cannot. You cannot even build trust out of a stack of eloquently crafted words. Authoritative credentials, a title, or a letter of recommendation from a *big shot* may give you some credibility and get you to the interview. However, you still have to be believable to close the sale.

How do you make yourself more believable? First, you must make eye contact. Without good eye contact, the committee members may become suspicious of you and wonder what you are hiding. Be sure to smile. Don't become so self-involved and nervous that you forget to relax and smile. Smiling is infectious and will help you and the committee members relax. Also, use open gestures. Don't sit at the table with your arms folded tightly over your chest. Keep your arms and hands open, which will support the fact that you are an open-minded person. Use a firm handshake. There is nothing worse than a wet, sweaty handshake. Finally, have good posture and project a strong voice.

Interviewers are Bombarded with Visual Stimuli that Register at the Preconscious Level

From the moment we walk into the interview, we begin giving off a series of verbal and nonverbal cues. For example, do you walk into a room tall, or do you slump? Do you have a firm handshake? Do you refer to your patients as *legs* and *arms,* or do you refer to them by name? Do you refer to nurses as derogatory, or do you give them the respect they deserve as colleagues?

An enormous amount of communication is taking place as thousands of multichannel impressions get carried to the brain. Most impressions register at the preconscious level. As a result of the beliefs, the brain forms a continuous stream of emotional judgments and assessments: Do I trust this person? Is she honest, evasive, threatening, or friendly? Is he interesting, boring, warm, cold, or anxious? Is she confident, insecure, or perhaps hiding something?

The emotional judgment that forms in your preconscious mind about the speaker determines whether you will tune in or tune out their message. If you distrust someone at the emotional level, little of what that person says will get through.

Getting to Trust

How do we use our natural self to reach the emotional center of our listeners? **First, you've got to be believed to be heard.** When dealing with the ADCOM, trust and believability are synonymous. You can't have one without the other. To communicate effectively with the committee, they must trust you. And to win their trust, you must be believable. Belief occurs at the gut level; it's acceptance of faith, emotionally based, and bypasses the intellect.

During the interview, each committee member sifts through your nuances of behavior. For example, does your voice quiver, or does it project authority? Do your eyes flicker hesitantly or gaze unflinchingly? Is your posture confident or timid? These nuances of behavior speak the language of trust.

People learn as babies who they trust and why. One day my son Eddie and I were at the airport on our way to Orlando, Florida, where I was to present a seminar. While sitting in the chairs by our gate, a toddler playfully strolled over to us with a big smile on her face. She was cooing and drooling and having a grand old time. Eddie and I played peekaboo with her, causing her to shriek with laughter and excitement. Then she suddenly strolled over to a man sitting next to us and smiled playfully at him. Without saying a word, he gave her a look that said, "I'm not interested in you, little girl. Go away"! The little girl's face went from a huge smile to a bit of pout. She ran from the man and knew that he represented trouble; he wasn't safe.

You cannot communicate with a baby using words. Instead, infants relate to facial expressions, energy, and sound. A baby responds with the same set of verbal cues. The smile is the language of our emotional centers. Even a baby knows that a person who doesn't smile lacks warmth and safety. We learn early in life that the people we should trust are those who (genuinely) smile. To communicate effectively, we must relearn the language of trust.

Did you ever meet someone and instantly like or dislike that person but not know why? When you meet someone for the first time, the emotional center in your brain receives thousands of nonverbal cues that register at the preconscious level. Your intuition comes from this; you form an almost immediate impression of that person. You develop an image that is detailed and often richly colored with emotion.

Most candidates approach the interview as though their essay, grades, and GRE scores count most. They fail to realize that the individual committee members don't comment on logic and reason when they leave that interview. Instead, they typically say, "I like her," or "I don't believe him," or "There's something about her that I like."

Some people can naturally do this without understanding how it works. The candidate who knows how to speak the language of the brain's emotional center—the language of trust—is the candidate most likely to be believed and accepted. That language communicates very rapidly and effectively.

The Likability Factor

In 1984, President Reagan ran for reelection against Walter Mondale (most of you probably weren't born then). A Gallup Poll examined three areas concerning each candidate: (1) issues, (2) party affiliation, and (3) likability. On the issues, the candidates were considered dead even. Mondale, the Democrat, clearly had the edge when it came to party affiliation. Concerning likability, however, Reagan had the advantage and won the election. Again, it was the personality factor that dominated.

As applicants, we pride ourselves on having an outstanding grade point average, test scores, and years of hands-on medical experience. But when it's time to interview, it's your likability that determines whether you receive a letter of acceptance or a letter of rejection. As soon as you walk into that interview room, it's the visual connection that sets the beginning of trust and believability.

The Eye Factor

The eye is the only sensory organ that contains brain cells. Memory experts invariably link the objects they remember to a visual image. Research shows that it's the visual image that makes the most significant impact in communication.

In the 1960s, Professor Albert Mehrabian pioneered the understanding of the effectiveness of the spoken message. He looked at three factors relating to the spoken message:

- The *verbal* message, or the actual words that we use, is what most applicants concentrate on, but this is the most insignificant part of the spoken message.
- The *vocal* component comprises the intonation, projection, and resonance of your spoken message.
- The *visual* message. **However, the visual message, the emotion and expression of your body and face as you speak, carries the most weight.**

Professor Mehrabian also found that the degree of consistency or inconsistency among those three elements determines the believability of your message. The more the three factors harmonize, the more believable you are as a candidate. If your verbal message is not in harmony with your body language, you send a mixed signal to the emotional center of the other person's brain. Your message may or may not get through to the decision-making, rational portion of your brain. Mehrabian quantified the three components of the spoken message as follows:

- The verbal component   =   7%
- The vocal component   =   38%
- The visual component   =   55%

In other words, what you see is what you get. If you come into the interview room yawning or dressed inappropriately, nothing you do or say will help you. The interviewer is likely to shut you out immediately and not hear a word you have to say.

HOW DO YOU ENHANCE YOUR MESSAGE?

Eye Contact

The first way to enhance your communication is with eye contact. Making eye contact is the number-one skill you should develop before you interview. Three rules and exercises for maintaining eye contact follow:

Rules

1. Use involvement rather than intimacy or intimidation.
2. Count to five (involvement), then look at the next interviewer; if you are in an interview with three committee members, be sure to make eye contact with all three while answering the question. Use the 5-second rule above.
3. Don't dart your eyes; this represents a lack of confidence.

Exercises

1. **Use video feedback**—tape yourself speaking with someone and watch for your use or violation of the three rules.
2. **Practice one-on-one**—Have a conversation with someone you trust and ask that person for direct feedback concerning the rules.
3. **Practice with a paper audience**—Draw smiley faces on sticky notes and then place them on a chair and practice making eye contact, counting to five, and looking to the next face.

Posture and Movement

The following way to enhance your message is with posture and movement. A good posture commands attention, and action shows confidence. Walk into the room, standing tall. Don't slump. When you speak to your interviewer, don't be afraid to add movement to your message. You don't have to wave your hands all over the room, but use open gestures to come across as a friendly, open-minded person. Four rules for posture are as follows.

Rules

1. Stand tall.
2. Watch your lower body; don't lean back on one hip or rock back and forth.
3. Get in the ready position; lean slightly forward if you're sitting or on the balls of your feet if you're standing.
4. Use movement to show that you're excited, enthusiastic, and confident.

Exercises

1. Walk away from the wall.

   Stand with your back against a wall, heels pressed against the wall along with your head, neck, and shoulders. Try to push the small of your back into the wall. Now simply walk away from the wall and feel how upright and correct your posture becomes. Try to shake off this posture; you can't. Practice this exercise daily so that when you walk into the interview room, you'll command attention.

2. Use the ready position.

   Remember, if you're standing, sit up slightly on the balls of your feet. If you are sitting, lean slightly forward toward the interviewer.

Dress and Appearance

The third way to enhance your message is with dress and appearance. You get only 2 seconds to make your initial impression on your interviewers. If you blow it, it may take more than 30 minutes to recover, and most interviews last for only 20 minutes. So, it is critical to make a powerful first impression.

When you dress up for an interview, only 10% of your skin should show. Be sure that your face is well shaven or your makeup is not too overbearing. Comb or style your hair, avoid wearing extravagant jewelry, clean and trim your nails, and use cologne or perfume sparingly.

Rules

1. Be appropriate—*When in Rome.*
2. Be conservative; when in doubt, dress up.
3. Men, always button your jacket.
4. Use perfume and cologne sparingly.
5. Always bring a small mirror and check your face and teeth before interviewing.

Exercises

1. Get feedback. Ask friends and relatives to assess how well you present yourself. Be open to constructive criticism.
2. Be observant; read fashion magazines. Find a style with which you are comfortable. Don't go over the edge, however.

Gestures and Smile

The final way to enhance your message is with gestures and your smile. Do you speak with conviction, enthusiasm, and passion? Are you friendly or stuffy? Do you talk with open gestures and a warm smile, or are you a fig-leaf flasher, always covering and uncovering your groin with your hands? (a common nervous tick)? Remember, openness equals likability. So here are three rules for gestures and smiling:

Rules

1. Be aware of nervous gestures and stop them.
2. Lift the apples of your cheeks—smile. Make believe that you have apples on your cheekbones and try to lift them to your forehead.
3. Feel your smile, but beware: phony smiles don't work.

Exercises

1. Imitate someone whom you feel is an effective communicator and play the part with gusto. Get used to using open gestures and expressions.
2. Be natural. Incorporate some of these gestures into your daily communication.

THE ENERGY FACTOR

Energy is the fuel that drives the car of success. You don't want to run out of gas when you're halfway up the hill. Instead, think back to the last morning that you awoke refreshed like you could conquer the world. Wasn't that a powerful feeling? That place is where you need to be on the day of the interview—in the zone. This section focuses on ways to unlock your inner energy and present yourself in the best light to the ADCOM.

Voice and Vocal Variety

Use intonation and inflection in your voice. Speaking in a monotone can be deadly and can put your listeners to sleep. Instead, observe and practice the following rules and exercises to add energy to your voice.

Rules

1. Make your voice naturally authoritative; speak from the diaphragm.
2. Put your voice on a roller coaster; practice reading from magazines using intonation and inflection.
3. Be aware of your telephone voice; it represents 84% of the emotional impact when people can't see you.
4. Smile when talking on the telephone; people can feel your smile right through the phone.
5. Put your real feelings into your voice.

Exercises

1. Breathe from the diaphragm. Take in a deep breath from your nose and let it out slowly, stopping to feel the pressure on your diaphragm. Speaking from the diaphragm is where a strong voice originates.

2. Project your voice. Try speaking in a normal voice first, and then project your voice, so it reaches the back of the room. Try to find the correct depth in your voice without straining your vocal cords.

3. Practice varying your pitch and pace. Watch reporters on the network news, as they are masters at using vocal variety. Notice how they emphasize certain words to draw you into the story.

Words and Nonwords

Energize with words and avoid using nonwords that are meaningless and take away from your message.

Rules

1. Build your vocabulary, especially with synonyms.

2. Paint word pictures. Create motion and emotion with metaphors.

3. Beware of jargon, especially medical jargon. Say "operating room" instead of "OR."

4. Avoid meaningless nonwords like *ah* and *um*, or words used to stall like *so*, *well*, and *you know*. Replace those words with a silent pause. An adequately timed pause adds drama, energy, and power to your message. Try listening to the voice of the famous commentator Paul Harvey on YouTube (Again, I'm dating myself). He was the master of the pause and made a career out of using the technique. Since many of you will not know who Paul Harvey was, Google him or go to YouTube to find old recordings of his work.

Listener Involvement

Humans communicate, and books dispense information. Try using the following techniques to add an extra punch to your communication:

Rules

1. Use a strong opening. Make it visual and energetic by including pauses, action and motion, and joy and laughter.

2. Maintain eye communication. When you enter the room for a group interview, survey your listeners for 3 to 5 seconds, gauge, and adjust.

3. Lean toward your listeners.

4. Create interest by maintaining eye contact and having high energy.

Use Humor Effectively

President Ronald Reagan was the oldest president in history when he debated Walter Mondale in 1984. The moderator of the debate asked about Reagan possibly not having the stamina to be an effective president—he was 69 years old. The audience broke out in laughter, and those words changed the entire campaign in Ronald Reagan's favor. You can also Google that debate. Reagan anticipated the *age* question and prepared this witty response, which turned out to be the most talked-about sentences uttered at the debate.

I do not recommend telling jokes at your interview and remembering that fun is better than funny. The goal is not comedy but connection. Find the form of humor that works for you, and be natural. If you feel it's too risky, then avoid it.

Karin's Experience

Let's look at what one of my friends and colleagues says about her interview experience at Yale University. Karin Augur did not get accepted the first year she applied; however, she reapplied the following year with a different result after making some adjustments. Her experience offers a great deal of insight into the interview process and what she learned about herself as a person.

> Applying to PA school or any other graduate school can be a very stressful process. Knowing yourself and the profession you strive to enter are two essential factors in the application process, particularly during the interview. To be sure that a career as a physician assistant is what you truly desire, you must have an in-depth and intimate knowledge of what a physician assistant does. Conveying that knowledge and your passion for the profession to your interviewer will translate into a successful interview.
>
> When applying to PA school, an impressive application is always important. However, when you interview, demonstrating your attributes in person is even more critical. The interviewers are looking for someone with strong character, good communication skills, and focused goals. Therefore, even with mediocre qualifications on paper, an impressive interview can significantly increase your chances of being accepted.
>
> My first attempt at PA school proved to be a painful eye-opener. After graduating from one of the top five schools in the country, having earned a BA

in biology, I was convinced that earning a Ph.D. for a research career was my calling in life. However, after several months working in a cell biology laboratory, I realized this was not my life's dream.

I soon began volunteering at a university emergency department, where I first encountered a physician assistant. Immediately, I knew that career path was one that I would enjoy, and I began preparing to enter PA school directly. I filled out all of the applications and mentally began to prepare for the interviews. During that year of preparation, I also became engaged to my current husband and found myself preparing for a wedding. As you can imagine, the year was quite hectic and emotionally overwhelming. Then, one by one, I heard from each of the schools where I interviewed; all of them rejected me. I could not believe it. What had happened? After the initial shock subsided, I soon realized why I was not offered a seat in the class.

Despite being physically present at the various interviews, I was not present in spirit. Besides being distracted by my wedding plans, I had not fully let go of the idea of a research career. The following year, I not only had to deal with a bruised ego, but I also needed to take a long, hard look at myself. I continued doing research and volunteering in the emergency department. I decided to start shadowing a PA and realized I had more to learn about the profession. I quickly embraced the idea that, yes, I wanted to be a PA. I focused my energy on improving myself as an applicant. As a result, the following year, I got accepted to the school of my choice. I completed the program in two years, finishing second in my class.

Whatever your goals are in life, you must embrace them fully. During the application process, I learned to embrace my goals fully; I failed to do that the first year I applied. Understanding your strengths and weaknesses and improving upon them are excellent ways to make yourself a stronger applicant. Learning as much as you can about physician assistants and how you as an individual will satisfy your dreams is as important to your interview as it is to your lifelong happiness.

I think the take-home message in Karin's story is that you have to do some soul searching and ask yourself what your true motivation is for choosing this career path. So many applicants are just *testing the water*, as Karin did her first year applying. It wasn't until she did the work and realized that research was not for her that she could succeed. Karin is an Ivy League graduate with excellent GPA and test scores. She is also a brilliant and likable person. She received many interviews her first year applying, yet she was not accepted. Her twin sister (Kirsten), also bright and likable, was my classmate that year, and I know it was a significant hit to Karin's ego not to be in our class too. The fact is, although Karin looked great on paper, the interview committee saw that her commitment to become a PA was not strong enough. She did not sell herself as a motivated and passionate applicant that year.

SUMMARY

In summary, after reading these three interview chapters, you are now well-armed to *ace* your PA school interview. Remember to focus on qualities and multipliers when answering your interview questions. The ADCOM already knows the type of applicant they will choose, and you want to show them that you are their perfect applicant. Remember, *it's not about you; it's about them!*

Equally important is utilizing high-impact communication skills at your interview. The visual and vocal components of your message that day are just as important as the answers you provide. Be sure to dress appropriately, make eye contact at all times, smile, speak passionately, and use open gestures.

I would strongly recommend signing up for a *mock* interview before your actual interview. Doing a mock interview allows you to practice under fire and relieve some of that pre-interview anxiety. You will also learn what areas of the interview you need to improve. Many colleges offer mock interview services; however, they must understand the PA profession and what type of questions to ask you.

[CHAPTER 10]

Financial Aid

Now that you're going to PA school, it's time for a reality check relative to paying for your education. For example, you can expect to *invest* approximately $100,000 for your 2-year education. This number includes:

- Tuition
- Books, uniforms, and instruments
- Technology fees
- Food, board, transportation, and miscellaneous
- Health screen
- Background check
- Lab fees
- Student health fees
- Student medical insurance

THE ALL-IMPORTANT QUESTION: CAN I AFFORD TO GO TO PA SCHOOL?

In my opinion, the real question you should be asking yourself is: Can I afford *not* to go to PA school? If you are passionate about becoming a PA, then the answer to this question will be an easy one. I left Yale in 1994 with a little over $60,000 worth of debt, which is the equivalent of $111,936 in 2021. My starting salary in 1994 was approximately $45,000, which is equivalent to $81,000 today (consumer price index [CPI], BLS). However, the median salary for PAs (2021) is currently $115,390, or $55.48 per hour. The take-home message is that the wages for the PA profession are growing at a much higher rate than the average professions.

Even though the investment seems relatively high—it is just that—an investment. So it would be best if you thought of this investment in terms of what your return on investment (ROI) will be. For instance, according to the National Association of Colleges and Employers (NACE), the average college graduate (master's degree) salary in 2021 is $50,944.

The average starting salary for a PA (2021) is approximately $90,000–$100,000, and depending on your specialty area, that number can be as high as $120,000 (BLS). So if you do the math, you can see that you will earn considerably more money as a PA than you would in most other professions requiring a graduate degree.

Let's look at the math, assuming an average starting salary of $90,000 for a PA and the average starting salary for other masters-level graduates. We will also assume that each profession receives a 3% raise per year. After 10 years, you'll be way ahead of the curve if you invest in PA school (Table 10.1).

Table 10.1. Comparison Between the Average Salary of a PA Professional and Other Master-Level Graduates.

Year	PA Profession	Other	Difference	
1	$90,000	$50,000	$40,000	
2	100,940	51,500	49,440	
3	103,968	53,045	50,923	$154,545
4	107,087	54,636	52,451	
5	110,299	56,275	54,024	
6	113,607	57,963	55,644	
7	117,015	59,701	57,314	
8	120,525	61,492	59,033	
9	124,140	63,336	60,804	
10	127,864	65,236	62,628	
Total:	**$1,123,445**	−573,184	= $550,261	

Note that your ROI for PA school occurs after 3 years. Also note, in 10 years, you will earn over one-half million dollars more if you choose the PA route. Finally, I would point out that I assumed the raises you would receive as a PA would be the same as for the *other* professions. In reality, a PA with 10-years' is very likely to earn much more than $127,000 at that point.

So the real question becomes, can you afford *not* to invest in PA school?

DECREASING YOUR INVESTMENT

Let's say that you plan on attending Duke's PA program and realize that the projected investment will be $87,036. Is there any way to reduce that investment or get reimbursed for your investment after you graduate? The answer is yes.

Let's look at the various expenses listed above. First, you will notice that there is only one way to reduce your costs while in PA school: food, board, transportation (including parking), books, and miscellaneous. The rest of the items are fixed costs that you cannot do much about.

Let's look at how you may be able to save some money, looking at each one of these items individually.

1. Tuition: You may qualify for reimbursement or a scholarship.
2. Books, uniforms, and instruments: You can buy used books and medical equipment online. The cost of uniforms will primarily include lab coats.
3. Technology fees: Nonnegotiable.
4. Food, board, transportation, and miscellaneous: I strongly advise sharing an apartment with one or two other students, grocery shop at large wholesale chains, minimize eating out, use public transportation to avoid parking fees, or live close enough to walk to school. Be sure to be mindful of all of your expenses and ask yourself: "Do I need this?"
5. Health screen: You may have this done by your primary care provider and covered by your insurance.
6. Background check: Nonnegotiable.
7. Lab fees: Nonnegotiable.

8. Student health fees: Nonnegotiable, unless you live in the same town as the program and your parents cover you.
9. Student medical insurance: May be negotiable.

HOW WILL I PAY FOR PA SCHOOL?

Now that we know that the investment for PA school can run in the six-figure range, you may be wondering: "How am I going to pay for this?" In this section, I will cover the various financial aid options.

What Is Financial Aid?

Financial aid is funds provided by federal, state, universities, or external agencies. There are also scholarships and grants (gifts) which require no repayment. In addition, the federal government provides student loans at low interest rates. The majority of students pay for their education with student loans.

The Application Process

The application process for financial aid starts with completing the Free Application for Federal Student Aid (FAFSA). The application can be found at FAFSA.gov and completed online. The FAFSA must be completed before you can be considered for federal, state, and university financial aid.

Since you will need tax return data to accomplish the form, I recommend using the IRS Data Retrieval Tool, which allows you to access the IRS tax return information needed to complete the FAFSA and transfer the data directly into the FAFSA application from the IRS website. This tool is the easiest way to provide your tax data, and it's the best way to ensure that your FAFSA application has accurate tax data.

What Happens Once the FAFSA Is Completed?

Once you complete the FAFSA application, your financial aid award letter will be determined and sent to the student financial services office (for each program), which may request additional information after receiving it. The programs will notify you by email regarding your eligibility for grants, scholarships, and federal loans. Review all of the information regarding your financial aid award, then either accept or reject the loans.

Federal Unsubsidized Loans

Securing a federal unsubsidized loan is the way most students will fund their education. Unsubsidized means that the loan's principal payments do not begin until after graduation, but the federal government pays the interest while in school. The student may pay the interest monthly while in school or defer the interest payments until after graduation. I recommend the former. If you postpone interest payments, the interest will accrue.

To qualify for a federal unsubsidized loan, you must complete the FAFSA application. On July 1, 2021, the **Federal Reserve raised interest rates for the 2021-22 academic year by nearly a percentage point:** 2.75% to 3.73% for Direct Subsidized and Direct Unsubsidized loans for under-graduates. 4.3% to 5.28% for Direct Unsubsidized loans for graduate or professional students. All students automatically qualify for these loans.

The maximum loan amount may vary yearly for graduate students. There is a great tool online at studentloans.gov, where you can access a repayment calculator based on the number of your loans. Although the standard time for repayment is 10 years, there are other options for more extended repayment plans.

Payment Plans and Loan Options

Your PA program may offer a monthly payment plan to pay part, or all, of your educational expenses. There are apparent benefits to begin making payments early, but this option will probably not be very realistic for most of you.

Some other loan options include private alternative loans from various vendors like Sallie Mae, Wells Fargo, Citizens bank, to name a few. These loans require a credit review and have variable or fixed interest rates. You can apply for these loans online, and you can make a side-by-side comparison at elmselect.com.

Federal graduate PLUS loans are another option. The interest rate for PLUS loans in 2021 is 5.3% (fixed). A PLUS loan is separate from the federally subsidized loans, but they are a good option for PA students. The student can apply for these loans online at studentloans.gov and receive approval in a matter of a few minutes. The Department of Education determines the loan amount, and your credit score will be a factor in the decision. You may use an endorser on these loans.

Tuition Reimbursement, Private Scholarships, and Other Sources

Some other sources of tuition assistance include private outside scholarships, local and national, which you can find on the program's website for a listing of available scholarships.

There are also federal grant programs like National Health Service Corps (NHSC), Indian Health Service (IHS), Department of Health and Human Services scholarships for health profession students from disadvantaged backgrounds, state programs, and through the American Academy of Physician Assistant (AAPA).

The National Health Service Corps is an excellent program covering tuition and providing you with a monthly stipend. You will incur a 2-year obligation to a designated (underserved) location. There are several sites throughout the country. You will be required to contact those sites for availability and negotiate a salary. The NHSC provides 400 awards each year. To qualify, you must complete a questionnaire and an application.

Contact information:

Contact: NHSC Scholarships
Division of Applications and Awards
5600 Fishers Lane, Room 8A-55
Rockville, Maryland, 20857
(315) 594-4400
Website: hrsa.gov

The IHS is another alternative. The IHS requires a minimum 2-year obligation in return for 2 years of financial support. Native American students have priority, but others may apply.

Contact: IHS Scholarship Office
(800) 962-2817
Website: ihs.gov

The Department of Health and Human Services also offers scholarships for health professional students from disadvantaged backgrounds. Applicants must be able to prove financial need and prove enrollment or acceptance to a PA program. Applicants must also be full-time students.

Contact:federalgrantswire.com/scholarships-for-health-professionals

There are some state programs available that include loan forgiveness. You will be required to work at a designated site in an underserved area and receive up to $20,000 in loan forgiveness.

It would be best to look into the Health Profession Shortage Area program, which provides loans at a dollar-for-dollar match for educational loans.

Many state/constituent chapters of the AAPA offer scholarship programs for PA students. Contact your state chapter for availability.

Veteran's Administration Military Benefits

The Yellow Ribbon GI Education Enhancement Program (Yellow Ribbon Program) provides the Post-9/11 GI Bill that allows veterans to attend private schools and graduate programs, costing more than the state tuition cap. Under the program, participating PA programs must offer a veterans-only scholarship which the VA will then match up to the total cost of tuition and fees.

For example, the Post-9/11 GI Bill will only provide $3,000 toward tuition/fees in the District of Columbia. George Washington University, however, the college to accept the WWII GI Bill, has signed up for the Yellow Ribbon Program and agreed to contribute $18,000 toward a veteran's tuition/fees. The VA will match that $18,000 contribution under the Yellow Ribbon Program. Thus, a veteran attending George Washington University will receive a full-ride toward their tuition and fees for up to $39,000/year.

Useful Resources

U.S. Department of Veterans Affairs: Post-9/11 GI Bill
https://www.va.gov/education/about-gi-bill-benefits/post-9-11/

U.S. Department of Veterans Affairs: Yellow Ribbon Program
(benefits.va.gov/GIBILL/yellow_ribbon/Yellow_Ribbon_Info_Schools.asp)

NAICU: Outreach to Veterans
https://www.naicu.edu/news-events/washington-update/2020/october-23/va-increases-oversight-on-gi-bill-useage

NAICU: About the GI Bill
https://www.naicu.edu/news-events/washington-update/2020/october-23/va-increases-oversight-on-gi-bill-useage

The individual PA program's financial aid office.

[CHAPTER 11]

Frequently Asked Questions

After being involved with coaching physician assistant (PA) school applicants since 1996, I have learned about some of the most commonly asked questions by PA school applicants. In this chapter, I am going to share these questions and provide the answers.

QUESTION #1: DO I HAVE A CHANCE?

Applicants routinely post this question on the PA Forum, along with their statistics (Grade Point Average [GPA], Graduate Record Examination [GRE], clinical experience), expecting people to respond with a yes? or a no? However, it is impossible to answer this question without reading the applicant's essay or evaluating their interview skills! A more appropriate question would be, "Am I a competitive applicant?"

The essay is your ticket to the interview, and a well-written essay can transcend less than average grades or medical experience. But, even then, if you make it to the interview and don't make that critical emotional connection with the committee, you will have no chance of being accepted.

So I advise applicants to stay focused and do the work necessary to become the perfect applicant before applying. Then I recommend writing a *killer* essay and learning how to *Ace* the PA school interview.

QUESTION #2: WHAT CAN I DO TO IMPROVE MY APPLICATION?

That's an easy question to answer.

First, forget about the published "minimum" requirements on a program's website. The perfect applicant will exceed the minimum standards for GPA, GRE scores, and health care experience.

Second, review Chapter 2 for real numbers from first-year "accepted" PA students. These are the numbers you should strive for because the competition will be bringing to the table.

Third, if you review the numbers in Chapter 2 and fall short in any area, work hard to improve your numbers before applying.

Finally, if you aren't a competitive applicant yet, consider waiting another year to strengthen your application before you apply. In the grand scheme of things, waiting one more year will not make a difference 10 years down the road. However, strengthening your application may also be the difference between getting into the PA school of your choice or settling for a school that you're not too excited about or where you may not be a good fit.

QUESTION #3: DO YOU HAVE ANY ADVICE FOR REAPPLICANTS?

Yes! The first thing the admissions committee (ADCOM) will do when they review your application and realize you are a reapplicant is to see what you've done to improve your application from last year.

Attempt to find out why you were not accepted last year. This may be hard to do sometimes, as you're likely to receive the standard response: "We had many competitive applicants this year, and unfortunately, we only have a limited number of slots available. We cannot accept everyone." This information is meaningless. The answer is not personal to you, and it doesn't help you prepare to improve your application for the next cycle.

If you made it to the interview and did not get accepted, chances are you did not interview well, and you will need to work on your interview skills.

In any case, there are several things that you must do to demonstrate to the committee (this year) that you are a serious, passionate, and motivated applicant:

- Continue to take upper-level sciences courses, and get As.
- Continue to gain hands-on medical experience.
- Continue to shadow PAs.
- Continue to stay current with the PA profession by frequenting the AAPA website and your state chapter of the AAPA website.
- Try contacting students from the program and getting a sense of the program's qualities in accepted applicants. What does the program value most?
- Review the program's mission statement, and be sure to make yourself a good fit for that program. For example, if the program values community service, get some volunteer experience.

You need to anticipate one question at your following interview; "What have you done to improve your application this year?" If you do the work mentioned above, you will come across as a motivated and passionate applicant. If nothing changes, nothing changes!
(The next chapter in this book is for reapplicants. However, it might not be a bad idea for all applicants to read this chapter too.)

QUESTION #4: HOW DO I GET MEDICAL EXPERIENCE? I'M A FULL-TIME STUDENT AND I DON'T HAVE MUCH FREE TIME

Let me be direct here. Figure it out! How will you handle a rigorous PA program if you can't work part-time and go to school full-time? Are you not able to multi-task? Are you not able to manage stress? Are you not motivated enough to get the necessary experience to become a competitive applicant? These are just some of the questions an ADCOM will consider if you apply to PA school with little or no medical experience.

Unlike young medical school applicants who are not expected/required to have direct patient contact hours, there's a different philosophy concerning PA school applicants. The PA profession is not an entry-level profession. Remember, the first PAs were former Navy corpsmen with 3 or 4 years of combat medical experience. Competitive applicants will have 2,500 to 3,000 hours of hands-on direct patient contact. So why would you think that you would be a competitive applicant without medical expertise?

PA school is not for the very young applicant, as it is challenging to acquire patient contact hours when you are in college, especially if you decide on this career path later on in college. The mean age of a first-year PA school student is 26. Of course, those applicants get accepted to PA school right out of college, but I would say these applicants are more the exception than the rule.

I don't mean to discourage the younger applicants from reading this book; I want to be realistic about the application process and what it takes to be competitive. However, those young but mature applicants seem to figure out a way to get the experience and get accepted.

QUESTION #5: HOW DO I FIND A PA TO SHADOW?

Great question! Shadowing PAs is a requirement for applying to PA school. How would you know that you want to become a PA if you haven't shadowed a PA? However, with the advent of Health Insurance Portability and Accountability Act regulations, it has become much more difficult for PA school applicants to find PAs to shadow. It is almost impossible at many hospitals.

Fear not! The best way to find PAs to shadow is by joining your state chapter of the AAPA, attending local meetings, and networking with PAs in your community. Most PAs are very willing to give back to the profession by allowing applicants to shadow them. We all had to find PAs to shadow, and we appreciate the need for you to have to do the same thing. If you can find a group of PAs that you can meet face-to-face and network with, you will have a much better chance of success than if you contact random PAs in your area.

Many state chapters of the AAPA also have lists of PAs willing to allow applicants to shadow them. Give the organization a call and see if they can help.

QUESTION #6: I HAVE A LOWER THAN AVERAGE GPA, WHAT CAN I DO TO BECOME MORE COMPETITIVE AS AN APPLICANT?

The chances are that if you have a low GPA after finishing undergrad, you would need to take a lot more classes to move your GPA into a competitive range.

When I served on the ADCOM, I looked more at the applicant's *trend* versus the absolute GPA number. So, if you have a lower than average GPA, begin taking some upper-level graduate science courses: genetics, chemistry, and physiology. Be sure to get As in those classes to demonstrate to the committee that you can handle the rigorous didactic phase of the PA program. On the other hand, if you take five or six science courses and do well, you may be able to compensate for your overall lower GPA.

QUESTION #7: WHO SHOULD I (IDEALLY) ASK TO PROVIDE MY LETTERS OF RECOMMENDATION (LOR)?

First, I always recommend looking at the program's requirements to see if they have requirements relative to referees. Typically, I would recommend that you obtain an LOR from at least one PA. The other two LORs should come from an individual who knows you well enough to comment, specifically, on the qualities you have that would be valuable as a PA school student and as a graduate PA. Usually, a professor, supervisor, or MD is appropriate.

Be sure to consider the person you are asking carefully. For example, suppose it's getting late in the Centralized Application Service for Physician Assistants (CASPA) application process, and you are missing one LOR to verify your CASPA application. Would you feel comfortable calling that person on the phone and asking them to get the LOR submitted ASAP? If the answer is no, don't select that person to write your LOR. It may be tempting to ask a *big shot* to write your LOR because you think her name will carry much weight with the program. However, her name will be meaningless if she fails to submit your LOR on time, and you don't feel comfortable calling her to get her moving!

QUESTION #8: HOW MANY PROGRAMS SHOULD I APPLY TO?

With the advent of the CASPA application, it is now easier than ever to apply to multiple programs by accomplishing a single online application. The more programs you apply to, the better your odds of getting invited to interview. But does that mean you should apply to 40 programs?

Absolutely not! From my observations, most PA school applicants apply to anywhere from 5 to 15 programs. You should select the programs you choose to apply to be centered on the fact that you are a good fit for that program, not out of convenience or because you want to use the *shotgun* approach.

QUESTION #9: IF I'M ASKED, "HAVE YOU APPLIED TO OTHER PROGRAMS?" BY THE ADMISSIONS COMMITTEE, HOW SHOULD I ANSWER?

This is a legitimate question and a concern of many applicants whom I work with on mock interviews. Many applicants fear that if they tell the ADCOM they've applied to several programs, that information will somehow diminish their chances of being accepted to that program. The fact is, if you are a serious applicant, motivated, and passionate about becoming a PA, you *should* apply to several programs.

If you admit to applying to only one program, the committee will question your motivation for wanting to become a PA. Why would you put all of your eggs in one basket if you're motivated to become a PA?

If you apply to only one program, like Duke, your odds of acceptance may be less than 1%! With those odds, you don't appear to be someone who cares if they get accepted or not. But, on the other hand, perhaps you're just testing the water?

On the other hand, if you apply to 40 programs, you will appear unfocused and desperate. What could be the common denominator between 40 programs? How will you explain why you've chosen the programs you have? What do they all have in common? Good luck with that one.

The bottom line is that you will not diminish your chances of acceptance if you tell the truth! ADCOM members have been doing this for a long time, and they know and expect applicants to apply to multiple programs.

QUESTION #10: WHAT IF THEY ASK AT MY INTERVIEW: "WHICH PROGRAM IS YOUR TOP CHOICE?"

This question can be extremely anxiety-provoking. What if the program you're interviewing with is *not* your top choice program? Do you lie and tell the ADCOM it is? It's never a good idea to lie at an interview, but you can put a positive *spin* on your answer.

Think about it a different way. The chances are that if you are at an interview, you probably haven't been accepted to your top choice yet unless the program is your top choice and the answer to this question is easy.

Technically, even if a PA program is not your top choice, it is your *only* choice during your interview. If you've been accepted elsewhere and are satisfied with attending that program, you wouldn't need to interview at another program. So you can honestly answer, this school is my top choice. Why? Because it is your only choice, right now!

QUESTION #11: HOW IMPORTANT IS THE SCIENCE GPA WHEN LOOKING AT POTENTIAL STUDENTS, AND, IF NOT PROVIDED ONLINE, WHAT IS THE MINIMUM OR RECOMMENDED SCIENCE GPA FOR STUDENTS TO HAVE?

Typically, the medical core or prerequisite GPA can sometimes paint a more accurate picture of the applicant's performance in the sciences. Many programs use an applicant's performance in prerequisite courses, especially upper-level biology and chemistry courses, to *predict* if the student would handle the demanding and rigorous PA curriculum. Many programs recommend that applicants have a 3.2 or higher prerequisite GPA to be competitive with the applicant pool. You will find the average prerequisite GPA for most programs to be between 3.4 and 3.6.

QUESTION #12: WHAT KIND OF MEDICAL EXPERIENCE IS PREFERRED, INCLUDING THOSE FROM THE LIST OF SUGGESTIONS ONLINE?

On average, most incoming students will have a certification as a certified nursing assistant, Emergency Medical Technician/paramedic, medical assistant (MA), physical therapy assistant, or phlebotomist. Programs prefer applicants to have paid experience, but many students accumulate their hours by shadowing a PA and a physician. Realize that not all PA programs accept shadowing to fulfill the clinical experience hours, but you will find that many programs strongly recommend shadowing in addition to paid hours.

Shadowing is a great way for applicants to get a feel for the role of the PA in clinical practice and help the applicant understand the role of the PA. I think most programs would say that the purpose of having clinical experience is precisely for the reasons listed above. Many programs list acceptable experience requirements on their websites.

QUESTION #13: IS RESEARCH RECOMMENDED FOR APPLICANTS, OR IS CLINICAL EXPERIENCE ENOUGH?

Research is not something most programs put a lot of emphasis on simply because the role of the PA is not research-driven. However, many PAs contribute to medical research, but the goal of most programs is to produce the best mid-level providers through clinically relevant teaching. This is where quality clinical experience before PA school is so beneficial. As a result, you may find that many medical programs emphasize research more than PA programs.

QUESTION #14: DO MOST STUDENTS TAKE OUT LOANS FOR TUITION? IS THERE ANY FINANCIAL AID AVAILABLE FROM THE COLLEGE OR FROM OUTSIDE OF THE COLLEGE?

I would estimate about 95% of students will finance their tuition, expenses for the program (equipment and books), and living expenses through student loans. No PA program will ever encourage students to have an outside job while attending PA school. Most programs do not allow students to work outside of school.

See the financial aid section in this book for various loans, grants, and scholarships options.

QUESTION #15: IS IT COMMON FOR POTENTIAL APPLICANTS TO TAKE TIME OFF AFTER UNDERGRADUATE SCHOOL TO ACCUMULATE CLINICAL EXPERIENCE?

Many applicants apply to PA school while in their senior year of college. Other applicants may take a couple of years to fulfill prerequisite requirements. If your preparation requires time off between graduation and PA school, especially to accumulate clinical experience hours, I strongly recommend taking time off. Clinical experience is essential to being a competitive applicant; this is especially true for younger applicants who may be fresh out of college and have no clinical experience.

QUESTION #16: WHAT ARE SOME OF THE MOST COMMON MISTAKES INDIVIDUALS MAKE WHEN APPLYING TO PA SCHOOL?

Here are five major mistakes:

1. *Writing an ineffective personal statement.* You must be able to communicate in your personal statement that you understand what you are getting yourself into—meaning you know the role of the physician assistant, how PAs benefit the health care system, and what experiences (clinically) have led you to believe that the PA profession is a good fit for you. One typical opening sentence for many applicants is that "I played with my dad's doctor's kit ever since I was five years old or read my mom's anatomy book... ." ADCOMs see this so often; the words are meaningless and unrealistic. Be unique. Make sure to have someone else read your essay before you upload it into your CASPA application. Having a typo or grammatical error in your essay could be the *kiss of death* for your candidacy.

2. *Selecting the wrong people to write your LOR.* Find three people who will provide you with GOOD LOR. I realize that it is impossible to predict what another person will write on your behalf, but make sure they can elaborate on your skills and potential as a PA. Believe it or not, some physicians submitted an LOR with only one sentence! See Appendix 5 for more detailed information.

3. *Not meeting all of the prerequisite requirements before applying.* Make sure that you meet all of the requirements for the program(s) to which you are applying.

4. *Not meeting the selection criteria.* Most programs have a minimum recommended overall GPA of 3.0 or higher, prerequisite GPA between 3.2 and 3.4, clinical experience requirements, and a GRE score of 297 to 300. Some applicants hope programs make exceptions for their past performance, low GPA, and test scores. With the number of PA school applicants applying each year, programs accept

those applicants who meet, or exceed, the selection factors. Why would a program settle for less?

5. *Applying too late.* Many applicants wait until October through December to start the CASPA application. Each year CASPA opens in mid-April for entry into the following year's class, so it is essential to begin as early as you can. As mentioned in the CASPA chapter, many programs have rolling admissions, so it's first-come, first-served at those programs. See Appendix 4 for a current listing of programs that utilize rolling admissions. Keep in mind this list is current as of 2021 and is certainly subject to change.

QUESTION #17: I AM A FOREIGN MEDICAL GRADUATE (FMG), WILL MY CLINICAL EXPERIENCE COUNT TOWARD A PROGRAM'S CLINICAL REQUIREMENTS?

Some programs count foreign MD hours toward their clinical experience requirement. So be sure to check with your program(s) before applying. Realize, however, that FMGs will still have to meet all of the academic prerequisites listed for each program.

QUESTION #18: IS THERE A PREFERRED MAJOR THAT WILL MAKE ME A MORE COMPETITIVE APPLICANT?

If you are in undergraduate school, I recommend choosing a biology or chemistry major if you know you will be applying to PA school. The reason for this is that you are likely to meet all of the prerequisite requirements for most programs by the time you graduate. Non-science majors may have a lot of catching up to do to acquire the necessary prerequisites.

Having said that, if you are a career changer and your major is not in science, it doesn't mean you cannot apply to PA school. You will need to take the prerequisites, and if you do well, you will be as competitive as any other applicant.

QUESTION #19: MY MOTHER IS A PA, WOULD THIS HURT ME OR HELP ME IN REGARD TO APPLYING TO PA SCHOOL?

Great question! I can't see how your mom being a PA would hurt your chances. If anything, her career as a PA should be a good resource for you to understand the profession better, and maybe she has recommendations on places to get your clinical hours. She's also *been there, done that* with PA school. She could provide excellent support as you go through PA school!

On the other hand, you will need to have your application and goal to become a PA stand on its own. Don't project a sense of entitlement, and be sure to express why *you* want to be a PA. You might come off as a bit immature if you cannot explain why you are choosing this path, and your answer better not be, "Because my mom is a PA."

QUESTION #20: I'M AN OLDER APPLICANT; WILL THAT HURT MY CHANCES OF ACCEPTANCE?

Never think that you are too old for PA school. Nontraditional students can bring a lot to the table. If you're going back to retake classes, be sure to do well in the prerequisite coursework. More than any other factor, the ADCOM wants to be assured that *any* applicant can handle the rigorous science coursework in PA school.

Additionally, programs are looking for specific qualities in applicants applying to PA school. However, those qualities are not necessarily relevant to the medical field, and many older applicants have the transferable skills needed to fulfill those qualities.

[CHAPTER 12]

Reapplicants

Winners never quit, and quitters never win

—Vince Lombardi

If you are one of those reapplicants who did not get accepted to PA school last cycle, or previous cycles for that matter, this chapter is for you. Rejection feels horrible, but give yourself a break. The fact is, only 31% of applicants get accepted each year to a PA program. Therefore, approximately 7 out of 10 applicants get rejected to PA school every year! Does that mean those other 31% of applicants are better candidates? Not necessarily. If you did not get accepted, chances are those who succeeded may be doing something different than you. Either something went wrong during the application process, or you scored poorly at your interview.

If you're worried about being a PA school reapplicant, you're not alone. While the process is still the same, the thought of reapplying to PA school routinely leads to anxiety. You may have heard admissions committees (ADCOMs) might view reapplicants less favorably, but that is not true.

Again, considering the statistics in the first paragraph, most applicants will be applying for the second or third time. Reapplying to PA school does not decrease your chances for the next cycle. It is how you prepare to improve your application that will make the difference this time around.

TIME TO REGROUP

After you've given yourself enough time to accept the fact that you didn't get accepted, and after you've got your wind back, it's time to regroup and begin your plan for the next cycle. First, take a deep breath and ask yourself, "Am I ready to do the work necessary to improve my application for the next application cycle?"

ARE YOU WILLING TO DO THE WORK?

Vince Lombardi once said, "Quitters never win, and winners never quit." Having helped thousands of applicants get accepted to PA school since 1996, I always preach about finding the motivation to succeed, finding *Inspirational Dissatisfaction*.

Inspirational Dissatisfaction is a concept I discovered a very long time ago in a best-selling book titled *Success Through a Positive Mental Attitude*, written by W. Clement Stone.

This philosophy means *I am so unhappy in my current situation that it is motivating the heck out of me to do something about it*. So, rather than becoming sad or depressed about your current situation, you become motivated by it, so inspired by it that you become willing to do whatever it takes to change your circumstances.

If you are undeniably determined to become a PA, you must be willing to take specific steps to prepare for the next cycle. Of course, some of you will have to do more work than others. Additionally, as you'll find out later in the chapter, some of you may have made one critical mistake that had nothing to do with your qualifications.

Let's first discuss those of you who did not get invited to the interview. I divide this chapter into two sections. Section 1 is for those of you who did not get invited to interview. Section 2 is for those who did get an interview but failed to get accepted.

SECTION 1: YOU DID NOT GET INVITED TO INTERVIEW

The first thing to consider if you did not receive an interview is *when* you submitted your application.

All programs publish an application deadline on their website or in their literature. Let's use the University of South Florida again as an example. This program's application deadline is October 1. However, a closer look reveals that the University of South Florida PA program utilizes *rolling admissions.* What does this mean to you? It means that if you waited until late September to submit your CASPA application, the class was likely already filled. Believe it or not, this may be the *only* reason you didn't get invited to interview. Please see Appendix 4 for a list of programs that currently utilize rolling admissions.

By definition, rolling admissions means that the program evaluates candidates' applications as they *roll* into the ADCOM. Strong applicants are immediately invited for an interview and accepted into the upcoming class if they're a good fit. The incoming class may be filled by May or June if the program utilizes this process. Therefore, the class is likely to be filled way before the application deadline. When did you apply?

I strongly recommend that all applicants submit their applications as soon as CASPA opens the cycle, typically in April. You may have a different result if you submit it earlier next time. Imagine if that was the *only* mistake you made?

Are You a Competitive Applicant?

If you submitted your CASPA application early but still did not receive an interview, you must be honest with yourself. For example, are you a competitive applicant?

During the soul-searching process of reapplying, you are going to have to take a hard look at where you may have fallen short. For instance, if you only met the *minimum* requirements for the programs you applied to last year, you were not a competitive applicant. Let's take a look at the University of South Florida's PA program to demonstrate this point (Table 12.1):

As you can see, *accepted* students exceed the *minimum* requirements significantly. However, if your Grade Point Average (GPA) and health care experience are closer to the minimum range, then you have some work to do.

Table 12.1. University of South Florida PA Program.

Minimum Requirements		Class of 2022 Accepted Students
Overall GPA	3.0	3.77
Science GPA	3.0	3.71
Health care experience	500 hours	2,209 hours

I understand you may not be able to raise your GPA significantly in a short period. However, you can start taking graduate-level science courses and get As. By taking more science courses and doing well, you show the committee that you are motivated to get into PA school and handle a rigorous didactic program. You should be aware that PA programs want to be reassured that applicants they accept will complete the program and pass the boards. (*It's not about you, it's about them.*)

I also recommend that you continue to gain health care experience, even if you already have a very competitive amount of clinical hours.

When I was on the ADCOM at Yale, my first question to reapplicants was; "What have you done to improve your application this year?" Some applicants don't have much to say, while others respond; "I've taken four graduate-level science courses and maintained a 4.0. I also gained another two thousand hours of medical experience."

What will your response be? Remember, *if nothing changes, nothing changes.*

REVIEW YOUR CASPA APPLICATION

The first thing you should do is print out a PDF copy of your previous CASPA application. Having a written application in front of you helps you review the entire application in its entirety. It will also provide the reviewer's perspective on how much time it takes to read an application.

I know you have only this one application to consider. However, please think about the CASPA review process from an ADCOM member's eyes. The reviewer will likely review tens, if not hundreds, of applications. As a former ADCOM member, I can tell you that reviewing applications is a serious time commitment and takes a lot of work. Your job is to make the reviewer's job easy. Unfortunately, sometimes applicants make the job too easy; a spelling error on your essay can rule you out quickly; attention to detail is an essential quality you need as a PA. Also, I often refer to using the title *Physician's Assistant* as the *Kiss of Death*. The committee expects that you know the correct name of the profession. I would often rule applicants out for this one mistake.

Next, be sure to read the application for any spelling or grammatical errors. I also recommend you have a friend or colleague check it too. Sometimes, when we stare at a document several times, we tend to miss errors that are obvious to a fresh set of eyes. I strongly recommend downloading the *Grammarly* app.

I am not going to cover the logistics of the entire CASPA application. Instead, I am going to list essential items that require your attention:

1. List *every* class you've taken for college credit.
2. Make sure your transcripts for every school are sent *directly* to CASPA.
3. Know your CASPA-calculated GPA.
4. Ensure Graduate Record Examination (GRE) scores (if needed) are shipped using the correct CASPA school code.
5. All of your documents sent to CASPA would reflect the updated information if your name changed.
6. Only include activities from the past 10 years at the college level or beyond.
7. Know the difference between health care experience, patient care experience, volunteer work, teaching, research, and non-health care experience.
8. Know the difference between full-time, part-time, per-diem, and temporary work.
9. Include a supervisor contact for each experience you list.
10. Always check *yes* to the question: "May we contact this organization?"
11. Letters of Recommendation are ready to go when the cycle opens?

Finally, your essay is the ticket to your interview. The essay is one of few things that you have any control over on your CASPA application. The PA school essay will probably be the most crucial piece of medical writing that you will ever accomplish. Don't treat the essay as another checklist item on your CASPA application. Start early; write several drafts; have a few PAs read your essay; then read it for content, grammar, and flow. Only after having done all these things will you be ready to submit your essay. Accomplish this process before the CASPA cycle even opens. And, yes, write a new essay for this cycle. Some of your past experiences won't change, but hopefully, you have more to add this time around. Again, utilize the *Grammarly* App for spelling and grammar review.

Some Other Questions to Consider if You're Not Invited to Interview
Can I reapply to the same programs?

Absolutely! As long as you've meaningfully improved your application from last year. Hopefully, you contacted the program to find out where you may have fallen short last time. At the same time, be honest with yourself about your stats and extracurricular background.

Should I wait an extra year before reapplying?

If you had a competitive application last cycle, there is no need to wait another year. However, if you need to accumulate a significant amount of clinical experience or take several classes to increase your GPA, you may want to wait an extra year.

Can I use the same letters of recommendation when reapplying to PA school?

The short answer to this question is yes. You can certainly use the same people to write your letter of recommendation. I would update any information that is appropriate from the last cycle.

Should I change my essay when reapplying to PA school?

Absolutely! I'm sure you've likely gained more health care experience, or you've taken additional classes. It is essential to include anything new in your essay. It would be a huge mistake to cut and paste your old essay into the new application.

SECTION 2: YOU DID HAVE AN INTERVIEW BUT WEREN'T ACCEPTED

If you received an interview, you likely met all of the criteria (on paper) the program looks for in applicants they choose to admit to their program. However, looking great on paper is not enough. You have to perform at the interview. Without a video of your interview(s) to analyze, it's difficult to know precisely where you may have fallen short. The following is a list of the most common errors applicants make during their interview:

1. They fail to dress appropriately. The proper attire to wear to a professional, graduate-level interview is a suit. There is no exception to this rule. Be sure to shine your shoes; groom facial hair; avoid too much makeup, perfume, flashy jewelry, visible body piercings, and wrinkled clothing.

2. They fail to make a solid first impression. Remember, first impressions take only *seconds*. If you fail to make a positive first impression,

it could take several minutes to recuperate. Most interviews only last for approximately 20 minutes, and you may not have time to recover in that period. Be sure to stand tall, smile, and give a firm handshake. A wimpy, wet handshake can instantly turn off the interviewer.

3. They fail to be *likable*. As mentioned earlier in this book, your interviewer(s) make their decisions emotionally and justify them with the facts. Failure to make that emotional connection with your interviewer is the most common reason why applicants get rejected. It doesn't matter how great you look on paper; you will undoubtedly get rejected if you aren't likable. Be sure to smile; make eye contact; use open gestures, inflection, and intonation in your voice; and monitor posture.

4. They are too wordy. Your answers should be brief and to the point. You will lose the attention of your interviewer(s) if your answers are long and drawn out. In order to give concise answers to interview questions, you need to prepare and practice, practice, practice.

5. They don't prepare for the interview. In my experience, many applicants struggle to answer the fundamental question; "Why do you want to be a PA?" Some applicants look like a dear in the headlights. It's as if they are shocked and surprised by the question. I don't care if you have a 4.0 GPA and 10,000 hours of health care experience; if you don't know why you want to be a PA, you will undoubtedly fall short. Therefore, I strongly recommend doing a *Mock Interview* at least once before each interview. Remember, *failing to prepare is preparing to fail.*

6. They let their guards down when not in the interview setting. They fail to realize the entire ancillary staff and the PA program staff are all evaluating you. If you are rude to the receptionist or any other applicants, you can ruin your acceptance chances. Treat everyone you meet that day as if they are the most important person in the world. Keep in mind that the ancillary staff works with each other every day of the year. They will not hesitate to report any rude or inappropriate behavior to their colleagues.

In summary, being a superstar on paper does not guarantee your acceptance into the upcoming class. It would be best if you made an emotional connection with the committee, and you came across as likable. The committee ultimately wants to know if you will be a good fit for the upcoming class.

Here are some key takeaways to prepare for the next cycle:

1. Develop Inspirational Dissatisfaction.
2. Apply early!
3. Compare your GPA and health care experience to the program's published *accepted students* statistics. Then, if you fall short, do the work to catch up!
4. Write a new essay.
5. Use the Grammarly app.
6. Reread the interview chapters in this book.

Remember, *if nothing changes, nothing changes.*

List of Postgraduate PA Programs

1. Albany Medical Center PA Post-Graduate Fellowship in Emergency Medicine
2. Albert Einstein Medical Center Physician Assistant Emergency Medicine Residency
3. Arrowhead Orthopaedic's—PA Orthopaedic Surgery Residency Program
4. Arrowhead Regional Medical Center—CEP America Paid Emergency Medicine PA Fellowship—Southern California
5. Bassett Healthcare Multispecialty—Surgical Postgraduate Physician Assistant Program
6. Baylor College of Medicine Emergency Medicine Physician Assistant Fellowship
7. Carilion Clinic Advanced Practitioner Fellowship in Orthopedic Surgery
8. Carilion Clinic Department of Emergency Medicine—Carilion Clinic Advanced Practice Clinician
9. Carolinas Healthcare System Acute Care/Critical Care Fellowship Program
10. Carolinas Healthcare System Primary Care and Urgent Care Fellowship: Pediatrics, Internal Medicine, Family Medicine, Urgent Care and Pediatric Urgent Care
11. Carolinas Healthcare System Specialty Care Fellowship: Cardiology, Urology, and Behavioral Health

12. Children's Hospital of Philadelphia—Neonatal Physician Assistant Program
13. Dartmouth—Hitchcock Medical Center Cardiothoracic Surgery Physician Assistant Post Graduate Residency Program
14. DMC Orthopedic Surgery and Sports Medicine PA Fellowship
15. Duke University Medical Center—PA Surgical Residency Duke University Medical Center
16. Emory Critical Care Center NP/PA Post Graduate Residency Program
17. EVMS Physician Assistant Fellowship in Emergency Medicine— Emergency Medicine
18. Hartford Healthcare PA Surgery—Critical Care Residency Program—Residency and Surgery
19. Hospital Medicine PA Fellowship at Regions Hospital
20. Illinois Bone and Joint Institute—Postgraduate PA Orthopedic Residency Program
21. Intermountain Medical Center Trauma and Surgical Critical Care—Postgraduate Fellowship for PAs and NPs
22. Iowa Emergency Medicine Physician Assistant Residency Program
23. Jane R. Perlman NP/PA Fellowship in Emergency Medicine
24. Johns Hopkins Bayview Medical Center—Emergency Medicine PA Residency
25. Johns Hopkins Hospital—Postgraduate Critical Care Residency for PAs
26. Johns Hopkins Hospital—Postgraduate Surgical Residency for PAs
27. Marquette University—Aurora Health Postgraduate Physician Assistant Emergency Medicine Program—Emergency Medicine Program
28. Mayo Clinic—Mayo Clinic Arizona PA Fellowship in Otolaryngology
29. Mayo Clinic Arizona Postgraduate Fellowship in Hospital Internal Medicine—with optional Hematology/Oncology and Critical Care Medicine Tracks
30. Mercer-Piedmont Heart Physician Assistant Residency in Advanced Cardiology
31. Methodist Debakey Heart and Vascular Surgery PA Residency Program—Methodist Debakey Heart and Vascular Surgery PA Residency

32. Montefiore Medical Center—Albert Einstein College of Medicine—Postgraduate Residency in Surgery for PAs
33. Montefiore Medical Center—Postgraduate Ob-Gyn Residency
34. Nationwide Children's Hospital Child and Adolescent Psychiatry Physician Assistant Postgraduate Training Program
35. New York Presbyterian Hospital—Weill Cornell Medical Center—PA Residency in Internal Medicine
36. Norwalk Hospital—Norwalk/Yale PA Surgical Residency Program
37. Regions Hospital—Emergency Medicine PA Residency Program
38. SJMH Residency in Cardiothoracic Critical Care
39. St. Joseph Mercy Hospital—PA Residency in Cardiothoracic Surgery
40. St. Luke's University Health Network—Critical Care and Emergency Medicine Advanced Practitioner (PA/NP) Fellowship
41. Staten Island University Hospital Physician Assistant Postgraduate Fellowship in Emergency Medicine
42. Team Health EMAPC Fellowship—Emergency Medicine
43. Texas Children's Hospital Surgery Physician Assistant Fellowship
44. The University of Texas MD Anderson Cancer Center—Postgraduate PA Fellowship Program in Oncology
45. UCSF Fresno Emergency Medicine PA Residency
46. UCSF Fresno Orthopedic Surgery PA Residency Program
47. University of Florida PA Surgical Residency Program
48. University of Iowa Carver College of Medicine—PA Residency Psychiatry
49. University of Kentucky—University of Kentucky PA Residency in Neonatology
50. University of Missouri—Post Graduate Acute Care Residency
51. University of Missouri Postgraduate Emergency Medicine PA Residency
52. UPMC Advanced Practice Provider Postgraduate Surgical Residency Program—Surgery
53. UT Southwest Medical Center at Dallas—Physician Assistant Urology Residency Program
54. WakeMed Health and Hospitals—PA Residency in Trauma, Critical Care, and General Surgery
55. Winthrop University Hospital—PA Postgraduate Surgical Critical Care Program

56. Yale New-Haven Hospital Emergency Medicine PA Residency Program

   Postgraduate PA Programs Website: https://appap.org/programs/postgraduate-pa-np-programs-listings/

The Tournament Draw Technique Format

Make a list of all the eight most important items you will need to accomplish before applying to PA school:

1. _____

2. _____

3. _____

4. _____

5. _____

6. _____

7. _____

8. _____

Now place those items in the first round of the chart below. Use the Tournament Draw Technique to come up with the winner: the first item you need to accomplish.

Round 1	Round 2	Round 3	Winner
1.			
2.			
3.			
4.			
			Winner
5.			
6.			
7.			
8.			

PA Programs' First-Time PANCE Rates as of 2021

ALABAMA

Program	Most Recent PANCE	Five-Year PANCE
Faulkner	TBD	
Samford	TBD	
University of Alabama, Birmingham	83%	89%
University of South Alabama	95%	96%

ARIZONA

Program	Most Recent PANCE	Five-Year PANCE
Arizona School of Health Sciences	94%	96%
Midwestern University (Glendale)	97%	98%
Northern Arizona University	94%	96%

ARKANSAS

Program	Most Recent PANCE	Five-Year PANCE
Harding University	97%	95%
University of Arkansas	89%	92%

CALIFORNIA

Program	Most Recent PANCE	Five-Year PANCE
California Baptist University	89%	92% (3 years of data)
California State University (Monterey Bay)	TBD	
Chapman University	100%	96%
Charles R. Drew University	91%	89%
Dominican University of California	100%	98%
Loma Linda University	94%	94%
Marshall B. Ketchum University	100%	100%
Samuel Merritt University	98%	91%
Southern California University of Health	91%	88%
Stanford University	100%	94%
Touro University (California)	96%	96%
University of California (Davis)	90%	88%
University of La Verne		
University of Southern California	86%	95%
University of the Pacific	100%	96%
Western University of Health Sciences	90%	93%

COLORADO

Program	Most Recent PANCE	Five-Year PANCE
Colorado Mesa University		
Red Rocks Community College	97%	97%
Rocky Vista University	TBD	
University of Colorado	98%	97%

CONNECTICUT

Program	Most Recent PANCE	Five-Year PANCE
Quinnipiac University	98%	99%
Sacred Heart University	97%	92% (2 years of data)
University of Bridgeport	100%	99%
University of Saint Joseph	100%	100%
Yale University School of Medicine	95%	97%
Yale University School of Medicine (Online Program)	89%	89% (1 year of data)

DELAWARE

Program	Most Recent PANCE	Five-Year PANCE
Arcadia University	98%	99%

DISTRICT OF COLUMBIA

Program	Most Recent PANCE	Five-Year PANCE
George Washington University	100%	99%

FLORIDA

Program	Most Recent PANCE	Five-Year PANCE
AdventHealth University	96%	92% (4 years of data)
Barry University	95%	93%
Florida Gulf Coast University	95%	95% (1 year of data)
Florida International University Herbert Wertheim College of Medicine	95%	88% (3 years of data)
Florida State University	86%	86% (1 year of data)
Gannon University		
Miami-Dade College	91%	92%
Nova Southeastern University Fort Lauderdale	94%	97%
Nova Southeastern University Fort Meyers	93%	97%
Nova Southeastern University Jacksonville	95%	94%
Nova Southeastern University Orlando	100%	99%

(*Continued*)

Program	Most Recent PANCE	Five-Year PANCE
South University Tampa	97%	95%
South University West Palm Beach	TBD	
University of Florida	98%	99%
University of South Florida	95%	86%
University of Tampa		

GEORGIA

Program	Most Recent PANCE	Five-Year PANCE
Augusta University	98%	98%
Brenau University	TBD	
Emory University	96%	92%
Mercer University	100%	98%
Morehouse School of Medicine	TBD	
South College (Atlanta)		
South University	91%	95%

IDAHO

Program	Most Recent PANCE	Five-Year PANCE
Idaho State University	93%	96%

ILLINOIS

Program	Most Recent PANCE	Five-Year PANCE
Dominican University of Illinois	97%	86%
Midwestern University Downers Grove	95%	98%
Northwestern University	100%	100%
Rosalind Franklin University	98%	99%
Rush University	100%	99%
Southern Illinois University	100%	100%

INDIANA

Program	Most Recent PANCE	Five-Year PANCE
Butler University	100%	99%
Franklin College	TBD	
Indiana State University	89%	94%
Indian University School of Health and Rehabilitation Sciences	100%	97%
Trine University		
University of Evansville	100%	100% (2 years of data)
University of Saint Francis Fort Wayne	92%	97%
Valpraiso		

IOWA

Program	Most Recent PANCE	Five-Year PANCE
Des Moines University	96%	98%
Northwestern College	TBD	
St. Ambrose University	100%	95% 4 years of data
University of Dubuque	91%	96%
University of Iowa	100%	100%

KANSAS

Program	Most Recent PANCE	Five-Year PANCE
Wichita State University	100%	100%

KENTUCKY

Program	Most Recent PANCE	Five-Year PANCE
Sullivan University	98%	93%
University of Kentucky	85%	93%
University of the Cumberlands	93%	94% (4 years of data)
University of the Cumberlands (Northern Kentucky)	TBD	

LOUISIANA

Franciscan Missionaries of Our Lady University	96%	98%
Louisiana State University (New Orleans)	96%	96%
Louisiana State University (Shreveport)	100%	98%
Xavier University of Louisiana	TBA	

MAINE

University of New England	93%	94%

MARYLAND

University of Maryland Baltimore/ Anne Arundel Community College	96%	100%
Frostburg University	TBD	
Towson State University CCBC-Essex	100%	92%
University of Maryland Eastern Shore	TBD	

MASSACHUSSETS

Bay Path University	100%	95%
Boston University School of Medicine	96%	99%

(*Continued*)

MCPHS University (Boston)	96%	97%
MCPHS University (Worcester)	88%	91%
MGH Institute of Health Professions	86%	91% 3 years of data
Northeastern University	98%	99%
Springfield College	97%	97%
Tufts University	100%	100%
Westfield State University	95%	95% 1 year of data

MICHIGAN

Central Michigan University	85%	94%
Concordia University	TBD	
Eastern Michigan University	93%	98%
Grand Valley State University	100%	100%
University of Detroit Mercy	92%	95%
University of Michigan-Flint	TBD	
Wayne State University	98%	99%
Western Michigan University	97%	95%

MINNESOTA

Augsburg University	100%	100%
Bethel University	97%	98%

(*Continued*)

College of Saint Scholastica	86%	86% 1 year of data
Mayo Clinic School of Health Sciences	TBD	
Saint Catherine University	100%	99%

MISSISSIPPI

Mississippi College	97%	94%
Mississippi State University-Meridian	TBD	

MISSOURI

Missouri State University	100%	98%
Saint Louis University	95%	97%
Stephens College	100%	100% 2 years of data
University of Missouri-Kansas City	90%	98%

MONTANA

Rocky Mountain College	92%	96%

NEBRASKA

College of Saint Mary	90%	91% 3 years of data
Creighton University	TBD	
Union College	100%	97%
University of Nebraska	100%	100%

NEVADA

Touro University (Nevada)	95%	93%
University of Nevada Reno	79%	79% 1 year of data

NEW HAMPSHIRE

Franklin Pierce University	88%	94%
MCPHS University (Manchester)	88%	91%

NEW JERSEY

Monmouth University	100%	98% 4 years of data
Thomas Jefferson University (New Jersey Campus)	97%	96%
Rutgers University	100%	99%
Saint Elizabeth University	TBD	
Seton Hall University	100%	99%

NEW MEXICO

University of New Mexico	88%	92%
University of Saint Francis	97%	94%

NEW YORK

Albany Medical College	98%	97%
Canisius College	TBD	
Clarkson University	86%	93%
Cornell University	89%	96%
CUNY School of Medicine	86%	88%
CUNY York College	91%	92%
D'Youville College	96%	96%
Daemen College	98%	97%
Hofstra University	100%	99%
Le Moyne College	96%	96%
Long Island University	97%	99%
Marist College	92%	96% 3 years of data
Mercy College	88%	90%
New York Institute of Technology	98%	98%
Pace University (Lenox Hill)	97%	99%
Pace University (Pleasantville)	90%	90% 1 year of data
Rochester Institute of Technology	100%	95%
Saint Bonaventure	TBA	

(*Continued*)

St. John's University	85%	92%
Stony Brook University	98%	97%
SUNY Downstate Medical Center	87%	89%
SUNY Upstate Medical Center	88%	96%
Touro College (Bayshore) and Nassau University Medical Center	100% (bay Shore) 93% (NUMC)	97%
Touro College (Manhattan)	100%	98%
Wagner College	100%	96%

NORTH CAROLINA

Campbell University	98%	98%
Duke University	96%	97%
East Carolina University	97%	99%
Elon University	89%	96%
Gardner Webb University	94%	96%
High Point University	100%	95% 4 years of data
Methodist University	100%	98%
Pfeiffer University	TBD	
University of North Carolina	94%	91% 3 years of data
Wake Forest (Bowman Gray)	98%	98%
Wingate University	96%	98%

NORTH DAKOTA

University of North Dakota	89%	92%

OHIO

Baldwin Wallace University	100%	100%
Case Western Reserve University	94%	97% 3 years of data
Kettering College	96%	98%
Lake Erie College	100%	100% 4 years of data
Marietta College	97%	97%
Mercy College of Ohio	TBD	
Mount St. Joseph University	TBD	
Ohio Dominican University	98%	98%
Ohio University	100%	98% 4 years of data
University of Dayton	100%	96% 4 years of data
University of Findlay	99%	100%
University of Mount Union	92%	96%
University of Toledo	100%	90%

OKLAHOMA

Northeastern State University	TBD	
Oklahoma City University	97%	94% 3 years of data

(Continued)

University of Oklahoma (Oklahoma City)	91%	93%
University of Oklahoma (Tulsa)	100%	100%

OREGON

George Fox University	TBD	
Oregon Health and Science University	98%	98%
Pacific University	95%	97%

PENNSYLVANIA

Arcadia University	98%	99%
Chatham University	96%	98%
DeSales University	99%	99%
Drexel University	97%	97%
Duquesne University	96%	93%
Gannon University	100%	96%
King's College	88%	95%
Lock Haven University	100%	97%
Marywood University	94%	96%
Mercyhurst University	96%	97% 4 years of data
Misericordia University	53% 3 years of data	86%
Penn State University	100%	100%

(Continued)

Pennsylvania College of Technology	95%	90%
Philadelphia College of Osteopathic Medicine	96%	98%
Saint Francis University	100%	98%
Salus University	100%	98%
Seton Hill University	95%	93%
Slippery Rock University	84%	91% 3 years of data
Temple University Lewis Katz School of Medicine	100%	100% 3 years of data
Thomas Jefferson University (East Falls Campus)	97%	96%
Thomas Jefferson University (Center City)	98%	99% 4 years of data
University of Pittsburgh	94%	95%
University of the Sciences	TBD	

PUERTO RICO

San Juan Bautista School of Medicine	TBD	

RHODE ISLAND

Bryant University	91%	95% 4 years of data
Johnson & Wales University	100%	98%

(*Continued*)

SOUTH CAROLINA

Charleston Southern University	96%	96% 1 year of data
Medical University of South Carolina	95%	96%
North Greenville University	83%	91% 2 years of data
Presbyterian University	TBD	
University of South Carolina School of Medicine	96%	96% 2 years of data

SOUTH DAKOTA

University of South Dakota	96%	93%

TENNESSEE

Bethel University	96%	94%
Christian Brothers University	91%	91% 1 year of data
Lincoln Memorial University	94%	93%
Lincoln Memorial University (Knoxville)	TBD	
Lipscomb University	TBD	
Milligan University	100%	100% 1 year of data
South College (Knoxville)	94%	96%
South College (Nashville)	TBD	
Trevecca Nazarene University	98%	99%
University of Tennessee Science Center (Memphis)	90%	96%

TEXAS

Baylor College of Medicine	100%	98%
Hardin-Simmons University	100%	100%
Interservice Army Medical Center of Excellence	95%	95%
Texas Tech University Health Sciences Center	95%	96%
University of Mary Hardin Baylor	TBD	
University of North Texas Health Sciences Center (Fort Worth)	99%	100%
University of Texas Health Sciences Center at San Antonio	100%	100%
University of Texas Medical Branch at Galveston	97%	98%
University of Texas (Rio Grande Valley)	89%	92%
UT Southwestern School of Health Professions	98%	100%

UTAH

Rocky Mountain University of Health Professions	96%	97% 4 years of data
University of Utah	84%	93%

VIRGINIA

Emory & Henry College	86%	84% 2 years of data
James Madison University	100%	98%
Mary Baldwin University	100%	100% 3 years of day

(*Continued*)

Radford University	95%	97%
Shenandoah University	98%	97%
South University (Richmond)	97%	99% 2 years of data
University of Lynchburg	93%	97% 4 years of data

WASHINGTON

University of Washington	92%	92%

WEST VIRGINIA

Alderson-Broaddus University	88%	95%
Marshall University Joan C. Edwards School of Medicine	TBD	
University of Charleston	96%	95%
West Liberty University	TBD	

WISCONSIN

Carroll University	100%	97%
Concordia University	90%	97%
Marquette University	100%	100%
University of Wisconsin (La Crosse)	100%	100%
University of Wisconsin (Madison)	98%	98%

APPENDIX 4

PA Programs Utilizing Rolling Admissions (2021)

ALABAMA

Program	Rolling Admissions
Faulkner	Yes
Samford	No
University Alabama, Birmingham	No
University of South Alabama	No

ARIZONA

Program	
Arizona School of Health Sciences	Yes
Midwestern University (Glendale)	Yes
Northern Arizona University	Yes

ARKANSAS

Program	
Harding University	Yes
University of Arkansas	Yes

CALIFORNIA

Program	
California Baptist University	Yes
California State University (Monterey Bay)	Yes
Chapman University	Yes
Charles R. Drew University	Yes
Dominican University of California	Yes
Loma Linda University	Yes
Marshall B. Ketchum University	No
Samuel Merritt University	No
Southern California University of Health	No
Stanford University	Yes
Touro University (California)	Yes
University of California (Davis)	No
University of La Verne	No
University of Southern California	Yes
University of the Pacific	No
Western University of Health Sciences	Yes

COLORADO

Program	
Colorado Mesa University	Yes
Red Rocks Community College	No
Rocky Vista University	No
University of Colorado	Yes

CONNECTICUT

Program	
Quinnipiac University	No
Sacred Heart University	No
University of Bridgeport	Yes
University of Saint Joseph	Yes
Yale University School of Medicine	Yes
Yale University School of Medicine (Online Program)	Yes

DELAWARE

Program	
Arcadia University	Yes

DISTRICT OF COLUMBIA

Program	
George Washington University	Yes

FLORIDA

Program	
AdventHealth University	No
Barry University	Yes
Florida Gulf Coast University	No
Florida International University Herbert Wertheim College of Medicine	Yes
Florida State University	Yes
Gannon University	No
Miami-Dade College	Not Reported
Nova Southeastern University Fort Lauderdale	Yes
Nova Southeastern University Fort Meyers	Yes
Nova Southeastern University Jacksonville	Yes
Nova Southeastern University Orlando	Yes
South University Tampa	Yes
South University West Palm Beach	Yes
University of Florida	Yes
University of South Florida	Yes
University of Tampa	No

GEORGIA

Program	
Augusta University	Yes

(Continued)

Program	
Brenau University	Yes
Emory University	Yes
Mercer University	Yes
Morehouse School of Medicine	Yes
South College (Atlanta)	Yes
South University	Yes

IDAHO

Program	
Idaho State University	No

ILLINOIS

Program	
Dominican University of Illinois	Yes
Midwestern University Downers Grove	Yes
Northwestern University	Yes
Rosalind Franklin University	Yes
Rush University	Yes
Southern Illinois University	Yes

INDIANA

Program	
Butler University	No
Franklin College	Yes
Indiana State University	No
Indiana University School of Health and Rehabilitation Sciences	No
Trine University	Yes
University of Evansville	No
University of Saint Francis Fort Wayne	Yes
Valparaiso	No

IOWA

Program	
Des Moines University	Yes
Northwestern College	Yes
St. Ambrose University	No
University of Dubuque	Yes
University of Iowa	Yes

KANSAS

Program	
Wichita State University	No

KENTUCKY

Sullivan University	No
University of Kentucky	Yes
University of the Cumberlands	No
University of the Cumberlands (Northern Kentucky)	No

LOUISIANA

Franciscan Missionaries of our Lady University	Yes
Louisiana State University (New Orleans)	No
Louisiana State University (Shreveport)	Yes
Xavier University of Louisiana	Yes

MAINE

University of New England	Yes

MARYLAND

University of Maryland Baltimore/ Anne Arundel Community College	No
Frostburg University	Yes
Towson State University CCBC-Essex	No
University of Maryland Eastern Shore	No

MASSACHUSSETS

Bay Path University	No
Boston University School of Medicine	No
MCPHS University (Boston)	Yes
MCPHS University (Worcester)	Yes
MGH Institute of Health Professions	No
Northeastern University	No
Springfield College	Yes
Tufts University	Yes
Westfield State University	No

MICHIGAN

Central Michigan University	No
Concordia University	Yes
Eastern Michigan University	No
Grand Valley State University	No
University of Detroit (Mercy)	No
University of Michigan (Flint)	No
Wayne State University	No
Western Michigan University	No

MINNESOTA

Augsburg University	No
Bethel University	No

(Continued)

College of Saint Scholastica	No
Mayo Clinic School of Health Sciences	No
Saint Catherine University	No

MISSISSIPPI

Mississippi College	Yes
Mississippi State University (Meridian)	Yes

MISSOURI

Missouri State University	No
Saint Louis University	Yes
Stephens College	Yes
University of Missouri (Kansas City)	No

MONTANA

Rocky Mountain College	Yes

NEBRASKA

College of Saint Mary	No
Creighton University	Yes
Union College	No
University of Nebraska	No

NEVADA

Touro University (Nevada)	Yes
University of Nevada Reno	Yes

NEW HAMPSHIRE

Franklin Pierce University	Yes
MCPHS University (Manchester)	Yes

NEW JERSEY

Monmouth University	Yes
Thomas Jefferson University (New Jersey Campus)	Yes
Rutgers University	Yes
Saint Elizabeth University	Yes
Seton Hall University	Not Reported

NEW MEXICO

University of New Mexico	No
University of Saint Francis	Yes

NEW YORK

Albany Medical College	Yes
Canisius College	No

(*Continued*)

Clarkson University	Yes
Cornell University	No
CUNY School of Medicine	No
CUNY York College	No
D'Youville College	Yes
Daemen College	No
Hofstra University	Yes
Le Moyne College	No
Long Island University	No
Marist College	Yes
Mercy College	No
New York Institute of Technology	No
Pace University (Lenox Hill)	No
Pace University (Pleasantville)	Yes
Rochester Institute of Technology	No
Saint Bonaventure	Yes
St. John's University	No
Stony Brook University	Yes
SUNY Downstate Medical Center	Early Applications Encouraged
SUNY Upstate Medical Center	Yes
Touro College (Bayshore and Nassau University Medical Center	Yes
Touro College (Manhattan)	Yes
Wagner College	No

NORTH CAROLINA

Campbell University	Yes
Duke University	Yes
East Carolina University	Yes
Elon University	Yes
Gardner Webb University	Yes
High Point University	Yes
Methodist University	Yes
Pfeiffer University	Yes
University of North Carolina	Yes
Wake Forest (Bowman Gray)	Yes
Wingate University	Yes

NORTH DAKOTA

University of North Dakota	No

OHIO

Baldwin Wallace University	Yes
Case Western Reserve University	No
Kettering College	Yes
Lake Erie College	Yes
Marietta College	Yes
Mercy College of Ohio	Yes

(*Continued*)

Mount St. Joseph University	Yes
Ohio Dominican University	No
Ohio University	No
University of Dayton	No
University of Findlay	No
University of Mount Union	No
University of Toledo	Yes

OKLAHOMA

Northeastern State University	No
Oklahoma City University	No
University of Oklahoma (Oklahoma City)	No
University of Oklahoma (Tulsa)	No

OREGON

George Fox University	Yes
Oregon Health and Science University	Yes
Pacific University	No

PENNSYLVANIA

Arcadia University	Yes
Chatham University	No

(*Continued*)

DeSales University	Yes
Drexel University	Yes
Duquesne University	Yes
Gannon University	Early application advised
King's College	Yes
Lock Haven University	Not reported
Marywood University	Yes
Mercyhurst University	Not reported
Misericordia University	Yes
Penn State University	No
Pennsylvania College of Technology	Yes
Philadelphia College of Osteopathic Medicine	Yes
Saint Francis University	Yes
Salus University	Yes
Seton Hill University	No
Slippery Rock University	Yes
Temple University Lewis Katz School of Medicine	Yes
Thomas Jefferson University (East Falls Campus)	Yes
Thomas Jefferson University (Center City)	Yes
University of Pittsburgh	Yes
University of the Sciences	Yes

PUERTO RICO

San Juan Bautista School of Medicine	Yes

RHODE ISLAND

Bryant University	Yes
Johnson & Wales University	Yes

SOUTH CAROLINA

Charleston Southern University	Yes
Medical University of South Carolina	No
North Greenville University	Yes
Presbyterian University	Yes
University of South Carolina School of Medicine	Yes

SOUTH DAKOTA

University of South Dakota	No

TENNESSEE

Bethel University	Yes
Christian Brothers University	Yes
Lincoln Memorial University	Yes
Lincoln Memorial University (Knoxville)	Yes
Lipscomb University	Yes
Milligan University	Yes
South College (Knoxville)	No

(*Continued*)

South College (Nashville)	Not reported
Trevecca Nazarene University	Yes
University of Tennessee Science Center (Memphis)	Not reported

TEXAS

Baylor College of Medicine	No
Hardin-Simmons University	Yes
Interservice Army Medical Center of Excellence	Not reported
Texas Tech University Health Sciences Center	Yes
University of Mary Hardin Baylor	Yes
University of North Texas Health Sciences Center (Fort Worth)	Yes
University of Texas Health Sciences Center at San Antonio	No
University of Texas Medical Branch at Galveston	Yes
University of Texas (Rio Grande Valley)	Yes
UT Southwestern School of Health Professions	No

UTAH

Rocky Mountain University of Health Professions	No
University of Utah	No

VIRGINIA

Eastern Virginia Medical School	No
Emory & Henry College	Yes

(Continued)

James Madison University	Yes
Mary Baldwin University	Yes
Radford University	Yes
Shenandoah University	Yes
South University (Richmond)	Yes
University of Lynchburg	Yes

WASHINGTON

University of Washington	No

WEST VIRGINIA

Alderson-Broaddus University	Yes
Marshall University Joan C. Edwards School of Medicine	Yes
University of Charleston	Yes
West Liberty University	Yes
West Virginia University	Yes

WISCONSIN

Carroll University	No
Concordia University	Yes
Marquette University	No
University of Wisconsin (La Crosse)	No
University of Wisconsin (Madison)	No

Writing an Effective Letter of Recommendation

The purpose of the letter of recommendation (LOR) is to provide the admissions committee with a detailed description of an applicant's abilities and qualities, rather than to merely check off a box on the CASPA application.

Let's take a look at a sample LOR, then dissect it and point out the three key elements that make a great LOR.

Dear Ms. Dean:

Please accept this correspondence a strong recommendation for John Smith's application as a student in your physician assistant program. I am the current Dean of the College of Health and Human Performance at Mankato State University, and John was my student for 4 years and my teaching assistant for 2 years.

As a student, John was easily in the top 10% of his peers for 4 years in a row. John is intelligent, energetic, reliable, and above all he is a team player.

As my teaching assistant, John was rated the highest by more than 122 students who have taken my classes. He scored high in communication skills, knowledge base, and likeability. He proved himself to be a dedicated, hardworking, and diligent young man.

John also has a strong military background. He served for 4 years as a navy corpsman, and his experience in that position would provide great strength to his candidacy in your PA program, and as a PA in the future. He was also an air force officer, which explains his admirable ability to pay strict attention to detail.

This young man has a high social conscience, high energy, a cooperative style, and the uncanny ability to analyze complex problems in the health field in simple yet constructive context. His social graces are beyond reproach. John will make an outstanding PA. He really cares for people, and people care for him.

I strongly recommend John Smith for candidacy in your physician assistant program.

Sincerely,

Robert R. Rockingham, Ph.D.
Dean, College of Health and Human Performance
Mankato State University

CONTENT

This LOR contains three key elements of an appropriate and effective LOR:

1. Introduction and background of the writer
2. Writer's relationship to the candidate
3. Quantified claims rather than general statements

The purpose of the writer introducing himself in the opening paragraph is to qualify as a legitimate reference. It shows that the reference truly knows the applicant and can honestly and objectively comment on the applicant's achievements, interpersonal and organizational skills, communication skills, and so on.

Finally, the reference quantifies the applicant's claims. Many people make it seem like they can walk on water in their applications. If the writer uses "meaningful specifics" versus "wandering generalities," he or she lends more credence to the letter (e.g., "was rated highest by more than 122 students").

IDENTIFY CANDIDATE'S STRENGTHS

A powerful LOR does not simply recite the obvious: "Sue has a great GPA." It's quite obvious to the committee that Sue has a 3.7 GPA; it's on her CASPA application.

The writer should be more creative and spend enough time on the letter to make you stand out from the crowd. The writer is usually asked to evaluate the applicant in several areas:

- Academic performance
- Interpersonal skills
- Maturity
- Adaptability and flexibility
- Motivation for a career as a PA

The writer may comment on all of these areas or just a few. In the areas that the writer does choose to comment on, his/her comments should be specific and relevant to that area.

For instance:

- Academic performance: "Top 10% of his peers."
- Interpersonal skills: "He cares for people, and people care for him."
- Maturity: "A strong military background."
- Adaptability and flexibility: "The uncanny ability to analyze complex problems … in simple yet constructive terms."

FINAL THOUGHTS

1. Go back to the sample letter and highlight all of the qualities about John that are mentioned. Remember, "it's not about you, it's about them." The committee already knows the qualities that they are seeking in the perfect applicant and the more qualities that are mentioned in the LOR, the better fit you will be for the program.
2. It is very important to keep the letter short, concise, specific, and personal. If someone else's name can be substituted for yours without changing the content of the letter, it is too generic.
3. Be sure the writer is recommending you for PA school and not medical school.

Sample Essays

ESSAY 1: ATHLETE/EMT

Reproduced with permission from Laura P.

Some call them "pre-race jitters," but I call them the starting point of my journey toward a career as a physician assistant. They fully kicked in at the Penn Relays starting line as my heartbeat quickened and butterflies fluttered around my stomach in nervous excitement. I was soon grabbing the baton from my teammate, 100 meters behind the girl in first place. I gained little ground on her, and as I approached the last 200 m of lap two, nothing could stand in my way. I moved confidently, ensuring quick leg turnover despite the burning in my leg muscles. At 800 m, I handed off the baton, my personal best putting our team slightly ahead. A runner since the sixth grade, I became an expert at keeping my composure in stressful situations, persevering, and chasing my aspirations both on and off the track.

In addition to instilling the traits I need to be an effective physician assistant, the parallels between my favorite running event and the demands of a PA career reinforce that I am built physically and mentally for the PA profession. The 800 m race requires endurance and sprinting ability; I can run long distances, but my talent lies in stamina and speed. I thrived in the 800 m race, just as I prefer the challenge of working in a fast-paced, multi-faceted healthcare setting.

My time in a clinic undergoing physical therapy to recover from a hamstring tear affirmed my desire for a busy medical environment. More specifically, physical therapy spurred my interest in muscle injuries and recovery; I was fascinated that one wrong movement could result in sudden muscle injury. After physical therapy and shadowing, I realized that I wanted to play a more significant role than rehabilitation post-injury. I wanted to be part of a collaborative team that diagnoses and treats various medical issues, with autonomy to perform procedures and prescribe medications, yet continuously learn from physicians' expertise. I wanted to become a PA.

When I hit upon my dream career as a senior at Wake Forest University, I was ready to chase it. I immediately began earning my Emergency Medical Technician certification and sought opportunities as a research assistant and a clinical trial volunteer. During one strength training session, I watched an elderly patient with knee osteoarthritis jog an entire lap around the track, tears coming to her eyes as she revealed the widest smile I had ever seen. She was ecstatic to run and do so with lessened pain, overcoming an obstacle that once seemed impossible. After that, I knew I would always want to have a personal interaction with patients in my career, giving them hope and seeking to make a difference in their lives.

My experience serving my hometown as a volunteer EMT also enhanced my interest in patient care and pediatrics. On my first day, I watched as the paramedic dropped to her knees to the young patient's level, asking softly, "Hey bud, what happened?" before explaining that the blood pressure cuff would give his arm a quick hug as mommy does. I admired the paramedic's ability to put the child at ease and noted the importance of empathetic communication and meeting patients where they are.

As a CHOP ED medical scribe, I learn something new about pediatric care during every shift. I remember listening to the physician speak with a 3-year-old and her mother as she asked how the little girl was hurt. I wrote, "Mom notes patient was running at a public pool, mom pulled patient toward her by a forearm to scold her, patient immediately cried and refused to bend L elbow." While listening to obtain the remaining history, I moved down to the medical-decision-making section and typed "History consistent with Nursemaid's elbow." In the plan section, I wrote, "4:00 PM. I will perform elbow reduction. Will prescribe Tylenol," and prepared a reduction procedure note. I knew there was likely no fracture, and thus, no X-ray would be ordered. Before the doctor started the physical exam, I anticipated the diagnosis and treatment plan based on the physician's first question. The physician's explanation to the mother confirmed my analysis, reminding me that proper diagnosis and treatment depend on asking the right questions. I enjoy the diagnostic process and continue to perfect my listening skills while expanding my medical vocabulary and knowledge of conditions ranging from respiratory distress to scabies to fractures.

In both my experience as a medical assistant in a plastic surgery practice and the PA shadowing program at the Hospital of the University of

Pennsylvania, I have noted the importance of holistic patient care, considering the mental, emotional, and physical aspects. I am eager to deliver excellent care to patients as a PA with a perspective informed by my competitive running background, interest in sports injuries, and experiences as a clinical trial assistant, EMT, scribe in a fast-paced pediatric environment, and medical assistant. Ready, Set….

ESSAY 2: LIFE-CHANGING EVENT/ FAMILY EXPERIENCES

Reproduced with permission from Kerri Mayo.

The life I built since I started working at the World Trade Center in 1999 was shaken from its very roots by the September 11 attacks. Something greater than myself orchestrating life placed me a few blocks away from my office at WTC on the day of the attacks. Five days from the incident was my wedding, and soon after, my husband and I moved to Portland, Maine, to start a new life. Since then, we had to work hard to build a comfortable life for our family. The priorities of life had to shift from my personal dreams to the dreams of my family. After working for a software company for 3 years, I took time off in 2005 to take care of my children. In 2008, I joined Maine Medical Center (MMC)'s Purchasing Department and was promoted to Maine Health, the parent company of MMC, as a lead analyst to implement an Electronic Medical Record, for MMC. Even though I was proud of my contributions, it was mostly the financial concerns that anchored me to the field. I was constantly frustrated with the limitations of my services.

One Summer evening, after decades, I was sitting alone in my living room. I had no more household chores or parental duties left to fulfill. The wheel of motherly concerns had stopped for a moment. My kids were away at a summer camp for the first time. The tranquility of the house gave me enough space to think about my individual goals. I realized my children would lead their own paths someday and I wanted my job to be more than a means to an end. It should be something I am passionate about. Nearly 20 years in the field of Information Technology confirmed me that IT is unable to give me the satisfaction of hands-on community service. My passion was healthcare, and I was determined to pave a way into the field with the time and various family responsibilities I had.

I chose to start volunteering at a local detox and worked with patients every week for the next 4 years.

I was drawn to the work as I was providing guidance and hope, lifting the spirits of countless addicts and alcoholics. I had finally found the field I wanted to invest my time in, medicine. I began researching programs offered in my area and was drawn to Physician Assistant, which provided a professional title to the work I was passionate to do. Further research and shadowing of PAs, RNs, and Nurse-Practitioners proved that I should base learning on the medical model. I hired a PA coach to guide me through the transition and started shadowing PAs while enrolling in Southern Maine Community College to fulfill the prerequisites.

My progress in completing courses was interrupted by the financial needs of my family. I rejoined MMC as a Project/Systems Analyst in a surgical center. It was a blessing in disguise as I was able to spend time in the Operating Room, helping others, that reinforced my decision to become a PA. Each day at work was a confirmation that I wanted to pursue this career.

Despite the financial pressures of supporting two children in a middle-class community, I became a Medical Assistant at the Maine Transplant Program to gain clinical hours. My role was to support patients in the pre-transplant phase. I attended daily morning huddles as an intricate member of the treatment team. Ordering all pre-cardiac testing, following up with dialysis units to prep patients, making sure their monthly labs were drawn, ensuring proper matches when a kidney was available, facilitating the pre-transplant classes, and answering patient-questions were included in my duties. My communication and people skills were immensely useful in building trust with patients during these daily encounters. Meanwhile, I started the remaining coursework and continue to date with a 4.0 post-baccalaureate GPA.

Amidst all my achievements, I see how hard it has been on my family to support me on my path. It is one of my goals to show my children that a worthy goal in life is worth making sacrifices for.

ESSAY 3: MOVED TO US AT A YOUNG AGE

Reproduced with permission from Sahar J.

I remained a patient of my pediatrician, Dr. Jenkins, until I was 20 years old. Although I did not realize it at 8, or even 18 years old, I do today:

Dr. Jenkins embodies everything I believe a health care provider should be. His genuine curiosity made me feel special as he inquired about all areas of my life whether they be prominent—about school, work, and family/friends—or what seemed trivial at a young age—his distress about my calcium levels due to my aversion to milk. Dr. Jenkins earned my trust, because I knew he cared about my health. He individualized me. He also inspired in me a secret dream; one I did not dare speak aloud: to become a health care provider myself one day.

Since elementary school, I carried my ambition in silence, because women from my culture do not dare to dream of education, independence, or autonomy. Knowing no English, each of my parents fled to America in the midst of the Iranian Revolution as teenagers, charged with the care of younger siblings and cousins. Compared to my ancestors, women who were deemed unworthy of education, who married men they had never met and bore babies when they were still children themselves, I recognize how lucky I am that my parents have encouraged both me and my sister to earn college and graduate degrees. I am a first-generation American, and I feel deep gratitude for the life my parents struggled so hard to give me. My gratitude, however, has a flip side: a debt.

For years, I paid that debt of gratitude by complying with my parents' wishes. Amongst the sacrifices I made to repay this debt, one that resonates is acquiescing with their wish to stay home and attend University of California, Irvine. Having both been forced to relinquish all childhood innocence when they fled to America—being burdened with responsibilities that some adults don't even carry, such as child care and financial hardship—it is evident why my parents resist autonomy for their children. Despite my independence already feeling threatened, I believed my only choice was to abandon my personal aspirations and succumb to their wishes. That meant becoming a civil engineer like my dad and living at home until I was deemed old enough to transition from my parent's jurisdiction to that of a Persian man's.

With this application, I am claiming a right that no woman in my family has claimed before—to take agency over my life. It wasn't until college that I discovered the field of Physician Assistants. Initially, it all seemed too good to be true: program duration, opportunity for lateral mobility, flexibility of the workload, quality of life, purpose. Because they have less administrative responsibility, PAs have extra time to devote to patient care. After meeting with, shadowing, and now working alongside PAs, I have witnessed career aspects that could be considered drawbacks: required physician supervision, rigorous recertification, occasional lack of patient trust, but I know without a doubt this profession and I are an ideal match and it would be the ultimate privilege to be a part of the PA community.

Although the primary purpose of a patient's visit is medical treatment, for many, especially those whose lives are comprised of ceaseless hospitals and doctors, little things make the biggest difference. Being exposed to a medical environment on a daily basis can desensitize one to the common qualms felt by patients. Acts of compassion like inquiring about a patient's weekend, holding a patient's hand during a biopsy, or sitting with a patient's silent pain after relaying an unsettling diagnosis, because of Dr. Jenkins, were always imagined to be obligatory. After now working in multiple healthcare environments, I have learned that they are not. Rather they are often a few of the many distinguishing qualities between a good, great, and extraordinary provider. Working in both a clinic and hospital setting has exposed me to a plethora of practitioners, each encompassing unique strengths I hope to accumulate as they all synthesize the kind of provider I aspire to be: confident, compassionate, curious, and trustworthy. My greatest joy is when a patient asks my physician, "What's that MA's name? I want to thank her." Becoming a PA will entrust me with a platform conducive to achieving my goal of providing people with the same dignity Dr. Jenkins afforded his patients. To treat everyone as the individuals they are, each with his or her own background, personality, challenges, triumphs, and story. Because everyone has a story.

My mother's story is that she dreamed of becoming a dentist. Instead, she got married, had children, and today works as a biller in a dental office. I have learned from her story and from my own, I was wrong. Living out parents' expectations will not repay the debt of gratitude felt. I am not my mother, nor am I any of the women who came before me who were denied the right to dream. My parents fled to this country to give me the opportunities I have today. Seizing those opportunities is the only way I can truly thank them.

ESSAY 4: PHYSICAL THERAPY BACKGROUND/FAMILY TRAGEDY

Anonymous

In my role as a Physical Therapist Assistant (PTA), I provide advanced wound care including a complete wound assessment, debridement, education, and dressing selection. I have been fortunate enough to have the luxury of spending quite a bit of time with my patients due to the nature of wound care and the often-extensive dressing changes. Mr. J is an example of one of those patients. Mr. J is a 57-year-old African American male with multiple medical problems, including diabetes, peripheral artery disease, and chronic kidney disease. Our team received a wound care consult for him regarding left foot osteomyelitis and a non-healing full-thickness wound. While establishing a rapport with Mr. J during a prolonged sharps debridement, I became aware that he had low health literacy, and his only family support lived out of state.

He joked about how he had a sweet tooth and told me he ate Little Debbie's daily. He did not understand how to control his blood sugar or the impact that hyperglycemia had on wound healing and his overall health. Along with his physical struggles, Mr. J also confided in me the mental distress he experienced due to caring for himself without any family support. I was able to offer written education and provide him with a few supplies, but I often wonder about Mr. J and how he got along after his discharge from the hospital.

As a PTA working in acute care, I treat numerous patients like Mr. J. These patients are the reason I have a desire to provide a more advanced level of care. Throughout my years working in healthcare, I have discovered I have a greater passion for the diagnoses, prognosis, and treatment of illness. I deeply wish to expand my knowledge beyond wound care and rehabilitative medicine. Becoming a PA will afford me with an education that covers a broad range of medical diagnoses and allow me to practice medicine in multiple disciplines. I use the patient example of Mr. J because I believe he embodies who the average patient in small town America is today. I have spent the past 8 years providing physical therapy and wound care services to patients in a regional hospital where the vast majority are low socio-economic status with low health literacy. Due to my personal background, I hold the ability to relate to these patients on a deeper level than simply providing a healthcare service.

I grew up in a low-income, single parent household. I had no education on health and how to take care of myself. I watched my mother battle depression over the death of my adolescent brother. I could have been on a path to becoming another Mr. J, except for one medical professional that changed my course. One of my first interactions with a physician assistant was with Heather, a PA at my primary care doctor's office. I saw her for many years for everything from strep throat to my annual exam. I admired her expansive skill set and appreciated the time she took to educate me. Even though she had a busy schedule, she never seemed rushed to get out of the room and I always left her office fully informed. Her kind demeanor appealed to me, as my main desire as a patient was to be heard. In retrospect, it was Heather that first sparked my interest in becoming a PA. Although I am no longer under her care, she made a lasting impression on me. She was the type of healthcare provider I aspired to be.

Being raised in a blue-collar family, I watched the people around me work hard for everything they had. I knew I wanted more for myself than what I had experienced. At that age, earning an associate degree was my idea of ultimate success. As a first-generation college student, I lacked guidance in choosing a career and obtaining a college education. I struggled with undiagnosed depression which made finding success that much more difficult. Returning to school as a more mature adult has been a very different and positive experience. I knew that pursuing PA school would be a long and challenging road. However, I have grown personally and developed the ability to learn and implement effective coping skills. While I did have to withdraw from courses after a car accident and my father's death, I am very proud of my more recent academic achievements. My academic progression exemplifies the type of student I truly am.

My interactions with patients, encounters with physician assistants, and life experiences have all woven together to form my decision to go to PA school. I aspire to play a bigger role in patient care and have the ability to diagnose and treat medical conditions. My experience medically and personally allows me to provide a comfortable environment for all patients. It is my life's passion to serve in the medical field at an advanced level and becoming a PA will enable me to do this.

ESSAY 5: INTERNSHIP IN A FOREIGN COUNTRY

Reproduced with permission from Tara Marie Pianko.

George's leg was black like tar, dripping in the scent of death. "Gangrene," Dr. Rahib informed me as he turned back to George and began to speak with him in Swahili, the native language of Tanzania. The fear in George's eyes was evident and required no interpretation. Dr. Rahib was attending to George's case and was my preceptor during my internship at Iringa Regional Hospital. He explained that George was suffering from an untreated wound as result of a motorbike accident—one of the leading causes of injury in Iringa. George's leg looked like the end of a burnt match stick and I was stunned. "Why did he wait so long to get treatment?" I asked as I began to undress part of his wound. Dr. Rahib explained that Tanzanians avoid medical care due to a shortage of doctors, the expense of treatment, and simply due to the lack of healthcare education in the area. Because of this George was at risk of losing his whole leg, or even his life, if Dr. Rahib didn't amputate below his knee. After relaying this to George, tears forged their way through the dust on his face and I reached for his hand, trying to offer him some sense of comfort. After I prepped George's wound, we brought him into the surgical suite for the amputation and I was careful not to let him see the hand-saw that was waiting to carve through his tibia and fibula. "Kumi, tisa, nane, saba…" George courageously recited as he counted back from 10 in Swahili until the anesthesia began to take effect. It was only after George closed his eyes that I let go of his hand and Dr. Rahib reached for the hand-saw. Over the next 30 minutes, I witnessed a lifesaving medical intervention that not only changed George's life forever, but mine as well. It was at this moment a seed was planted within me that made me want to devote myself to working directly with and helping patients like George.

Several years had elapsed since my unforgettable experience with George and I went on to study infectious diseases and bioterrorism at Georgetown University. With the events following 9/11 and the real threat of bioterrorism, I felt these studies combined my passion for science, problem solving, helping others, infectious diseases, and emergency medical intervention. In addition, I obtained my Emergency Medical Technician certification. Soon thereafter, the U.S. Food and Drug Administration (FDA) offered me a position as an Investigator. This was very intriguing and seemed to be a role that I would be challenged in. As an FDA Investigator, I have a mission to keep the public safe by identifying and mitigating intentional and unintentional risks associated with infectious diseases. However, as exciting as this role is, I soon found out that something important was missing—a sense of fulfillment like that I experienced as an intern in Tanzania. It was because of this that I knew a lifelong career at the FDA would not be my destiny, and it was during this time that kismet in the form of a sprained ACL brought my calling into clear focus.

While playing in a volleyball league, I sprained my ACL and the next day I was treated by a Physician Assistant (PA). Her confidence in handling me and her mastery of skills she demonstrated was incredible. A revelation occurred throughout my treatment with my PA as I reflected back to the experience with George and the effect he had while

I was in Tanzania—I want to be a healthcare provider who is attuned to the holistic needs of my patients. I began to research the PA field, interviewing every PA I had encountered. I found that the PA profession has a high degree of personal interaction with patients combined with the ability to critically listen, emphasize, and deliver care that makes a difference. I continue to affirm this through shadowing and volunteer positions. These experiences have shown me that being a PA would allow me to make a difference in direct patient care. Learning, diagnostic skills, and empathy, coupled with a willingness and ability to not only listen, but to hear, is as critical to quality health care as medical expertise; and these are the collective qualities I see in the PA community. This experience and sense of fulfillment brought me directly back to George and has led me to conclude unequivocally, that this is what I will be—a Physician Assistant.

I will strive as a PA to interact with those in medical need as people first, who happen to be patients as well, delivering the best care possible. My journey to this career commitment has taught me valuable lessons in time management, oral and written communication skills, teamwork, and maturity. I value my collective experiences and know they will help make me be the best PA one can be as I join such a diverse pool of medical providers. Reflecting to that epiphanic moment and the effect George had on me in Tanzania, I am grateful.

ESSAY 6: FOREIGN MEDICAL EXPERIENCE/SERVICE

Reproduced with permission from Makena Fowler.

Clinica de Adolescentes, a small hospital that made a huge impact. Seven days interning in this hospital in Quito was all it took to solidify my desire to pursue the physician assistant profession. Each day varied but one patient stood out. When her name was called, she came to the office door and anxiously took a seat on the child-sized bed in the hospital's only patient room. This patient was 12 years old and was seven months pregnant. Contraceptive care is not easily accessible in Ecuador, and it sees the highest rate of teen pregnancies in all of South America. During my week in the hospital, I saw many young women who were afraid, alone, ill-prepared, and financially unable to bring a child into the world. I also saw many women endanger their lives and the lives of their unborn children through self-inflicted abortions. Watching the doctor weigh his options between doing what was best for the patient and adhering to cultural customs revealed a new side of medicine. I realized that I want to spend my life advocating for these patients.

As a PA, I want to advance conversations on ethical medical dilemmas and work to find solutions that preserve cultural beliefs and boundaries while also providing safe medical care. Through this experience, I also learned that these dilemmas are not easily solved and that we may never find clear black and white answers. But I know that I want to spend my career striving to blur these lines, to be receptive to all sides of the story, and to take my patients' best interests to heart.

Hippocrates said it well: "Wherever the art of medicine is loved, there is also a love of humanity." My love of medicine and human connection began in high school as I enrolled in medical terminology and anatomy courses. I realized then that I wanted to pursue a career in healthcare. I volunteered in a clinic in high school, and while in college, decided to apply for a position as a medical assistant in my hometown.

I started working for PeaceHealth in a per diem position where I had the chance to work directly with MDs, NPs, and PAs. Through my experiences with each of these medical professionals, I found my perfect fit with PAs. I was drawn to the smaller portal, which allowed the PA to spend more time building a relationship and a community with their patients. I truly admired that the PAs were able to establish practices that value the individual from many different aspects of health and wellness, from emotional wellness to physical wellness to spiritual wellness. These characteristics stood out to me and I loved that, as a PA, I would be able to spend more time with my patients to truly understand their wellness needs and how I can assist them from a practitioner standpoint

In an effort to better understand my future patients, I spent my college career in the classroom studying chemistry, Spanish, and kinesiology while committing my time outside of the classroom to interning in hospitals in Latin America, working for my local hospital, and volunteering to serve CASA and other community organizations. In pursuing my goal of becoming a health care professional and advocate, I have learned the importance of building a supportive community and establishing a welcoming environment for the individuals we work with. I believe this starts with valuing each person's individualities. Every person has something unique to bring to the table, and with all the pieces of a community, we can build a stronger whole.

I have poured myself into my community because I desire to serve a wide population of individuals with public health as a primary goal.

Interning abroad, job shadowing, and working have all led me to the decision that the PA path is the right path for me. I thrive in the team-based environment that is created between physicians and PAs, and I would love the opportunity to continue to grow in my knowledge through collaborating with a physician as well as the opportunity to continue my education in the form of specialties. I have shadowed practitioners from general surgery, pediatrics, plastic surgery, neonatology, obstetrics, and internal and family medicine and I am fascinated by the opportunity to learn more about each of these specialties.

In my experience with direct patient care, I have heard many patient stories in which one health care practitioner has made all the difference. Quality patient care, medical ethics, community, continuous learning and adapting, and patient relationships contribute to this difference and are just a few of the reasons that I am pursuing a career as a PA.

Throughout my academic and professional career, I have strived to become a well-rounded health care provider. People do not easily fit into boxes. Patients come with emotions, traumas, accomplishments, experiences, and histories that make them who they are. Patients themselves are well rounded, and as medical professionals, we need to recognize this in order to effectively treat the whole patient.

ESSAY 7: CHILDHOOD TRAUMA/LOSS

Reproduced with permission from Mary Ishak.

My passion to pursue PA studies began when I experienced the devastating loss of my 43-year-old father from sudden cardiac death. I can recall the most traumatic night of my life, as tears were rolling down my face. Despite the chaotic environment in the emergency room, a woman, introducing herself as a Physician Assistant thoroughly explained the circumstances of my father's untimely death and offered her condolences. That moment ignited my passion of becoming a PA, because she radiated warmth and understanding in such a cold, sterile environment where my father was now missing. As I continue my volunteer and healthcare experiences, I know that I want to do something larger than that 13-year-old girl could have ever imagined.

I am fortunate enough to work as a Medical Scribe in both an emergency room and family practice setting. I have worked with Dr. Smith at her family practice, which allows me to learn how preventative medicine is the key to optimum health. My experiences as a Medical Scribe have provided me exposure to an extensive number of different patients, diagnoses, histories, and ICD-10 codes. These skill sets assisted me while visiting the villages of Guadalajara with my church.

A team of medical providers allowed me to communicate with natives about their lifestyle and counsel them in Spanish. My experience in Mexico has reminded me the satisfaction of empowering others to understand their medical conditions and make healthy choices. The opportunities I have to interact with patients are the moments that I truly see myself as a practicing PA.

I recall an interaction with an insulin dependent patient with renal disease. She became frustrated with her abnormal home glucose numbers, misunderstood the insulin dose, and medication regimen. The patient began to break down while I was taking her history, but when I sat down and talked to her, she collected herself. Under the supervision and direction of Dr. Smith, I printed an insulin sliding scale for her, hand wrote a medication list, and encouraged her onto a healthier lifestyle by incorporating her hobbies. She followed up with normal glucose readings and a sense of well-being. She hugged and thanked me for my patience and sympathy, and this patient centered approach will pave the way to decrease further risk factors from complications of diabetes.

There was an elderly patient following up on routine lab work, but during his appointment the patient was found to be in severe bradycardia. Dr. Smith instructed me to call 911 to arrange paramedic transport while the doctor called the emergency room. The patient. The patient became anxious and started crying, and so I validated his feelings, got him water, and accompanied him out to the ambulance truck. Our conversations are cherished because I was able to offer a glimmer of positivity and compassion for him during a stressful time.

There is nothing else I see myself pursuing, as it is the perfect combination of service and medicine. Becoming a successful PA will allow me to encourage patients onto a healthier lifestyle. The highlight of my workday lies in patient interaction, whether it is calming down a patient worried about their upcoming surgery, lending a listening ear, or sending urgent prescriptions to a nearby pharmacy. The ability to speak with diverse patients comes second nature to me, and there is excitement each day I walk into the clinic. Above all, understanding that every day I have an obligation to be there for a patient during their worst days of their lives.

ESSAY 8: RESEARCH/ HEALTHCARE OPERATIONS

Reproduced with permission from Atara S.

I am a natural caregiver. As one of ten children, I grew up helping to care for my five younger siblings. Needless to say, I quickly developed expertise in diaper-changing, dinner-cooking, and last-minute STEM-tutoring.

My upbringing fostered an interest in helping others. As an undergraduate at New York University, I studied Biology and Global Public Health. I pursued this double major to gain an in-depth understanding of both the scientific and societal issues underlying our most important public health problems and to contribute to their solutions. In classes on epidemiology, environmental health and health policy, I considered the ways in which I, as a citizen, can work within my local health and government agencies to not just treat, but to also prevent health challenges. For example, in a public health entrepreneurship class, I designed and pitched a survivor-led education program to promote awareness of sexual violence in colleges nationwide. My goal was to prevent assault on campuses in a personalized and effective way. I was passionate about this idea because I am driven to make a positive impact on the health and wellness of those around me.

During my sophomore and junior years, I volunteered at an NYU immunology lab. I researched lymphocyte trafficking and how levels of sphingosine-1-phosphate are altered when a virus infects the body because I believed in the project's potential to help create improved therapies for inflammatory diseases. More fundamentally, I wanted to support research efforts that would make a difference in the lives of patients.

I pursued my passion for patient-care after graduation by joining Care+Wear, a healthcare start-up based in New York City. Care+Wear creates innovative health wear, such as recovery bras for post-mastectomy patients, clinically accessible onesies for premature infants, and dignified hospital gowns with a covered backside. As a client relationship manager, I worked to expand the distribution network of Care+Wear products by building relationships with new and existing hospitals. In my role,

I interacted with patients across the healthcare spectrum on site visits, during product design, and when answering customer inquiries. I quickly found these encounters to be fulfilling and inspiring.

Eleven months after I joined Care+Wear, the company's mission became more personal to me when my father was diagnosed with stage 4 cholangio-carcinoma and became a Care+Wear customer. Throughout my dad's treatment, physician assistants played a central role in his care; as one of my father's advocates, I would often liaise with PAs who were both well-informed and empathetic. After each medical test, the PAs at Sloan Kettering invested the time to help us understand and digest the implications of my father's exams and how the results fit into the broader prognosis and treatment plan. Watching PAs work tirelessly to help my family cemented my conviction that I wanted to be a PA and touch the lives of patients through clinical work.

In order to have more direct contact with patients, I began working as a medical assistant in a dermatology practice in September 2019. Since joining the practice, I have accrued over 1,000 clinical hours, working alongside the office's physician and PA. In this role, I was struck by my ability to directly improve the lives of our patients. For example, in each Mohs procedure, I prepare the patients and inform them of what to expect. I assist the physician throughout the procedure and then educate the patients on how to treat the site until the next visit. From the first biopsy, to relaying the diagnosis, to assisting in the procedure, to recovery, I have had countless opportunities to directly influence the complete cycle of patient care. The closer I have gotten to patients, the more dedicated I have become to pursuing a future as a PA.

I believe that my experience in scientific research, healthcare operations, and direct patient care equips me to be a successful PA. I am well-informed about the requirements for a physician assistant and am excited for the opportunity to evaluate, diagnose, treat and educate patients. As a PA, I hope to utilize my degree to pay forward the kindness of PAs who treated my father and make a positive impact on each patient I encounter.

ESSAYS THAT DIDN'T WORK

Essay # 1:

My desire to pursue a career in medicine as a physician's assistant is a product of my professional and personal background, work ethic, and desire to positively impact others' lives. For the past 15 years, I have participated in chiropractic medicine, which has provided me with invaluable clinical experience in treating those ailments that respond to chiropractic medicine. Initially, it was the most rewarding endeavor of my life—the culmination of years of arduous schooling, clinical hours, and hard work. However, with that same clinical experience and professional growth, I became increasingly frustrated with the limitations of chiropractic practice and felt that something was missing. I was searching for a common thread in medicine, a more comprehensive vantage point that would allow me to treat a broader spectrum of medical conditions to help my patients. But, in my view, I saw a piece of the puzzle and not the entire solution.

Moreover, it was frustrating to have been educated in the medical model but to lack prescriptive authority. Ultimately, while I have enormous respect for chiropractic medicine as a means to an end, I became professionally disappointed and dissatisfied. This yearning to be a more complete healthcare practitioner led me to pursue a career as a physician's assistant.

Despite these philosophical concerns about my chosen profession, a recent life-altering experience ultimately fueled my passion for making the change: my mother was diagnosed with lung cancer. While following my mother's disease, I had the opportunity to meet her doctors and interact with them on a professional level. Their dedication and tireless pursuit of the best possible treatment inspired me and reignited my desire to pursue something more fulfilling. During this time, I became immersed in obtaining the best care possible for my mother, exhaustively researching the drug regimens and protocols best suited for her. Though it may sound a bit lofty, this personal mission further reinforced my belief that practicing medicine was my purpose in life.

In addition to my inspiration, I believe I have the right set of experiences to succeed in this field. Having practiced chiropractic medicine in inner-city neighborhoods for most of my career, I have developed patience, understanding, and compassion for working with people of different cultures and ethnicities—essential traits when working as a physician's assistant.

I feel that my passion, dedication, clinical experience, and maturity make me an excellent candidate for a program of your caliber. As an adult in my mid-forties and as a licensed chiropractic physician, I fully understand the commitment and stamina needed to meet the challenges of medicine, and I possess the academic requirements and critical thinking skills required to be an outstanding physician's assistant. I look forward to giving back as much as I know I will gain from the program and the profession, and I respectfully thank you for your consideration of my candidacy.

Comments:

This essay might have been acceptable if it weren't for the writer using the term "physician's assistant." The name of the profession is "physician assistant." Using the former shows a complete lack of knowledge about the profession and is what I call "The kiss of death" for an applicant. If I were reviewing this chart on the admissions committee, I would reject this applicant based solely on this critical mistake

Essay #2

The last few years have been a time for me to reflect, review my career objectives, and plan for change. I want a medical career with a promising future and direct involvement with people. My future career must meet my need for continuing education, provide an opportunity for change, and utilize my past life experiences, training, and skills.

The physician associate profession meets that criteria and the viability of the physician assistant profession are without question. The creation of a national healthcare system that demands affordable healthcare will only intensify the need for PA's, and indicators suggest that this profession will grow throughout the next decade and beyond. I still have 20 to 25 working years ahead of me, and I want my next career to be one that will offer both challenges and opportunities.

The role of the physician assistant goes beyond the symptoms and encompasses a deeper level of knowledge, compassion, and continuous learning. Of course, most effective healthcare professionals have empathy for their patients, along with the required skills and expertise. Still, a physician assistant makes a more significant contribution to my community and society.

For approximately 15 years, I have been practicing as a chiropractic physician, and I have established a reputation for providing high-quality care to my patients. I have communicated and coordinated care with primary care physicians and specialists in meeting patient's needs. Most referrals to my practice come from other healthcare providers. I attribute their confidence to my abilities as a team player and my understanding that a multidisciplinary approach is sometimes necessary. Having a family with small children made my decision to change careers difficult, but I feel it is best for my family and our future. Years of adjusting patients, including the strenuous activity associated with the physical therapy and chiropractic techniques I utilize in my practice, are beginning to take a toll on my body. I enjoy what I do, but my job is physically hard on me, and I don't want to lose my passion for helping people because of it.

The other compelling reason for choosing the physician assistant career is that the profession has made tremendous advancements in the medical field. But, unfortunately, we seem to have so many different philosophies and agendas that we have alienated ourselves from one another instead of growing stronger. My goal is to participate in a profession that will continue to grow, become an integral part of our healthcare system, and develop the essential tools and resources necessary to serve public needs best.

During my undergraduate years, I had to cope with my father's alcoholism. His disease affected our family, and my academic performance suffered because of that. My grades in Chiropractic College, however, reflect my level of maturity and my commitment to succeed. From elementary school through college, some of my extracurricular activities include my interest in music and my ability to play the Bouzouki, an ethnic Greek instrument. In addition, I formed a professional band that performed weekends at festivals, weddings, baptisms, and parties. To help finance my undergraduate education, I also owned and operated a hot dog concession stand during the summer months. In addition, I worked at numerous jobs with a variety of people. These experiences greatly enhanced my communication and social skills.

An effective physician assistant collaborates with supervising physicians while maintaining independence and nurturing a good rapport with patients. Therefore, my commitment to becoming a PA is unequivocal. During my career, I acquired the analytical, communication, and time management skills that will help me become a truly competent physician assistant, and I am confident that I will be an asset to the profession.

Comments:

In this essay, the writer makes several critical mistakes. First, he makes it all about "me." In the very first paragraph, he writes, "My future career must meet *my* need..." Remember my mantra throughout this book, *It's not about you; it's about them.* Second, this writer repeats the role of a PA throughout the essay. The reader of his essay is likely a PA, and certainly knows the role of the profession. Regurgitating this information wastes a lot of space he could use to write about more of his qualities. Third, in the fifth paragraph, the writer uses "we" as if he is already a PA. Finally, the writer doesn't answer the question as to *why* he wants to become a PA.

Essay #3

I knew I was meant for a career in medicine ever since an incident in the summer of 1990. Some friends and I were playing a little rough when Doris's toenail was accidentally ripped off. No adults were around, so despite the profuse amount of blood and Doris's hysterical crying, I knew we had to do something. Unfortunately, my fear and nerves were no match for my intense desire to help Doris, so I cleaned her wound and applied a bandage until her mom could get her to the doctor using a first-aid kit from my parent's closet. Doris will probably always remember that day as traumatic. Still, it was the day that I realized that practicing medicine was not just about vital signs and giving medication, but about giving patients the best care possible and peace of mind about their condition. I was hooked and knew that a career in medicine was my goal.

Upon my undergraduate graduation, I became an HIV/AIDS case manager in Camden, New Jersey. I worked closely with clients, families, social services, and medical professionals to coordinate services for people dealing with many life challenges. It was an invaluable experience that taught me to be empathetic and objective while focusing on the task at hand; I got up every morning ready to improve the health and wellbeing of my clients through care, compassion, and respect.

After serving as a case manager, I taught special needs students, providing daily instruction for them and tending to their basic medical needs. Because of my character and my passion for medicine, the school administration was confident in my ability to handle minor scrapes and bruises. Even parents of the most medically fragile students were comfortable with my first aid CPR training and my ability to react swiftly to emergencies.

While I gained valuable experience from serving as an HIV/AIDS case manager and working with special needs students, the most significant aspect of both positions was the deep awareness I gained of the healthcare disparities between the affluent and the underprivileged. In communities where needs are the greatest, educational resources and quality of healthcare are the weakest. I knew I wanted to make a difference by pursuing a career supporting physicians and serving urban communities.

I have innate and acquired skills that will make me a successful physician assistant, recognizing that the requirements go far beyond empathy and awareness of social injustices. I have been deemed a highly competent leader, organized and assertive, but not aggressive in other professional roles. I understand the competitive nature of the PA applicant pool; however, as a non-traditional student, I bring maturity, preparation, and confidence to my cohort. Since completing my bachelor's degree in psychology, I have completed upper-level science courses that have broadened my awareness and will help prepare me for a PA program. For example, in a recent genetics class, I researched the genetic disorder osteogenesis imperfecta. I learned about the delicate process a healthcare team undertakes when a mother with this condition delivers a baby.

I am prepared for a rigorous course of study and the practical experience that will lead me to a successful career as a physician assistant. I know what the job entails. I have had the opportunity to observe physician assistants conducting physical exams, diagnosing and treating illnesses, ordering and reading tests, counseling patients on preventive care, writing prescriptions, and empowering patients. I have seen how physician assistants must act as independent thinkers and doers while also consulting closely with supervising physicians, and I understand their role in a healthcare team. Moreover, my background as a case manager and public school teacher has prepared me to serve high-risk populations, aligning with my goal of helping urban communities.

I look forward to giving as much back to the profession as I know it will provide me with.

Comments:

This writer uses what I call the "lightning bolt" reason for choosing a career in medicine. He opens the essay with, *I knew I was meant for a career in medicine ever since an incident in the summer of 1990.* First, this incident occurred many years ago, and as a rule, writers should not discuss situations that occurred more than 10 years ago. Second, is it believable that a toenail injury shaped his vision for a future in healthcare at such a young age? I call this a "lightening bolt" moment because it's as if the writer was instantly called to medicine by this singular event.

Essay # 4

Several years ago, I had the opportunity to reevaluate my life plans. I realized I wanted to begin a career in the medical field and entered a medical assisting program. I learned of various medical professions during the training and became captivated by the physician assistant profession. I discovered it is one of the few medical professions that allows involvement in patient care and diagnosis and treatment.

At present, I work in a family practice office as a back office medical assistant and scribe. This job provides an opportunity to work alongside the doctor during each office visit. I add history, diagnoses, physical exam findings, and treatment plans to the electronic medical record for information that would be important to that particular visit. For example, when the doctor considers certain medications that may affect kidney function, I look to ensure the patient has no diminished kidney function on recent lab results. I question the patient and doctor for clarification, and I propose diagnostic tests or treatments for the doctor's consideration. Observing the doctor's ability to determine when a firm or compassionate hand is needed has also been highly enlightening.

I have also had to see the healthcare field from a patient's perspective. For example, a recent diagnosis of simultaneous ovarian and endometrial cancer has allowed me to see the difference a compassionate caregiver can make to a patient who is amid a severe diagnosis. It has also taught me the value of early diagnosis and treatment.

I currently live in a medically underserved rural area and understand many of the challenges. In particular, I recall one elderly diabetic patient who could not afford to drive a few miles to pick up his insulin at the office where I worked. I brought it to his tiny house on my way home. He also asked me for information on diabetic diets: I got a book to him the next day.

I prefer to work in family practice as a physician assistant to care for patients with varied conditions and backgrounds. I look forward to future challenges and rewards of a lifelong career as a physician assistant.

Comments:

The writer of this essay is very young, immature, and a bit idealistic. She mentions delivering insulin to a patient after work and then bringing a book on the proper diet for diabetes the next day.

She also implies that she practices medicine as a medical assistant. In the second paragraph, she writes, "*I question the patient and doctor for clarification, and I propose diagnostic tests or treatments for the doctor's consideration.*" I tend to doubt that she suggests tests and treatment options to her physician. Offering tests and treatment options to the physician implies she is his colleague with a medical degree. In the same paragraph, she uses the word "doctor" several times. I suggest using "physician" instead or at least alternating between doctor and physician. For some reason, I feel using "doctor" sounds a bit immature also. The distinction between the two words may be trivial, but to me, physician sounds more credible.

My last comment relates to the brevity of the essay. The writer is allowed 5,000 characters, and she only takes advantage of about half that many. Most applicants have trouble cutting their essays down to 5,000 characters.

Essay # 5

I have desired to be a physician assistant literally since the time I discovered what a PA is. Two things set in motion my dream of becoming a PA; First, I have had a desire since childhood to help people. The examples shown by both my grandfather and father as ministers were ever present influences on the desperate need of the human heart for healing, as well as the gratification that serving them and helping in the healing process can bring. My heart was stirred to help people-I went on various mission trips with my church to a Native American reservation and to Mexico and I witnessed the health needs of the people there, both physically and mentally. The secondary source of inspiration came due to meeting with and being treated by a PA at my doctor's office. Her personable and kind manner set me at ease and she was truly professional in her work. The initial encounter with that PA caused me to begin to investigate what was involved with becoming a physician's assistant. I shadowed two of the PAs that worked at my doctor's office, as well as a urologist who allowed me to assist in a supervised capacity in several surgeries. Even being given a small taste of the experience of assisting filled me with excitement and passion. The more I researched the role, the more intrigued and challenged I became, to the point of becoming the professional dream of my life.

The process of learning has always been, and will doubtless continue to be a source of great enjoyment for me. Because good grades had always come easily to me, I misjudged my natural academic strengths when it came to certain college-level classes. The mistakes I made related to overloading myself with class and work hours cost me dearly. While I did well, as a rule, my math and chemistry class struggles caused me to put my dream on hold, and I learned the hard way to succeed academically; I can never assume that a class is easy.

My study focus and efforts required a long hard look, as well as personal scrutiny. After reevaluating my time management and study techniques, I graduated with my master's degree in counseling psychology. Upon completion of my degree, I was required to pass a difficult exam to obtain licensure as a professional counselor and complete 3,000 hours of supervised experience. Since that time, I have been employed with Kingswood Pines Hospital for 3 years. While I enjoy interaction with people in their mental and emotional health needs, my dream of becoming a PA never died. In place of the discouragement I had toward becoming a PA, I began to see the strength of combining my ability as a counselor and being a PA as one final challenge I was ready to conquer.

With the encouragement of my family and professional colleagues, I felt encouraged to renew my dream of becoming a PA. Equally important to me was proving to myself as well as any school that I would attend that I can make good grades and successfully master the math and chemistry courses that stumped me before. Rather than taking short summer courses that stumped me before, I carefully and methodically planned my path to success. This meant returning to college and taking over not only the classes with undesirable grades, but also those in which I wanted to have a current and refreshed knowledge. Likewise, the chemistry classes were postponed until after I had spent a semester working individually with a tutor to ensure that I had a firm foundation and comprehension of the subject. Not only have I passed these classes but my grades were superior enough that the dean extended an invitation to join the honors program. My commitment is for this momentum to continue to spur me on to success throughout all remaining courses.

While nobody likes making mistakes or periods of uncertainty, I believe that my experiences have endowed me with more compassion and understanding than I could have had without them. In dealing with patients, I recognize that many of their health problems will likewise result from poor personal choices, but they are in no less need of my compassion. The listening skills and empathy I have cultivated in my practice as a counselor will only serve to embellish the care I hope to provide. Certainly, in my dealings with people, I have worked with various personalities many would initially view as challenging or off-putting, but my experience has sharpened my clinical judgment and increased my confidence and assertiveness. My approach will be one of humility, and born of a true appreciation to serve and care for others.

In keeping with this background, I feel that Baylor is the ideal choice for pursuing my education as a PA. After attending an information session, I was struck by the program director's words that he views the program as a finishing school of sorts, where the students are fine polished until they can shine. My desire is to reach my fullest potential, and this statement revealed to me that the faculty shares in that desire. While at a graduate level, the burden of academic success ultimately rests on my shoulders, it is encouraging to know that instructors will support and motivate me as well.

As a Texas resident, Baylor's name is a familiar one to me. Before learning the formal history of either the school, or the medical facilities, I was introduced to Baylor as a little girl when my grandfather underwent heart surgery in one of its Dallas-based hospitals. In college, I visited a friend at the Waco campus, and the animal lover in me was impressed and excited that they kept bears onsite! Also, as recently as last year, a dear friend of mine faced a life-threatening situation, and it was at another Baylor facility that she received the care she needed to survive.

On an academic level, Baylor impresses me as unparalleled. The ranking in U.S. News and World report as the nation's ninth leading PA program speaks for itself of the fine education and training its graduates receive. The rigors of a career as a PA demand a comprehensive and meticulous preparation period, and I believe that Baylor will best equip me to meet those demands.

I feel I can flourish in the role of a PA, and if I am fortunate enough to attend Baylor's program, I will do do so with the finest of education to support me. My determination has driven me to excel, my previous experiences have taught me that hard work has become my friend, and mediocrity a sworn enemy. The achievement of this goal will propel me to higher personal and professional heights and truly be the realization of a life-long dream.

Comments:

Whew! Where do I begin? First, the opening paragraph of this essay is way too long, has nothing in it to grab the reader's attention, and attempts to cram way too much information in a single paragraph. At a *minimum*, the writer needs to split this very long paragraph into two sections. Second, the first paragraph has multiple grammatical errors and use of the passive voice (more on passive voice following this essay.) Third, the writer also claims to have assisted the urologist in surgery while shadowing. Shadowing is watching, not doing. Fourth, assisting in surgery requires consent from the hospital and the patient. That would never happen! Some practices and hospitals don't even allow shadowing due to HIPPA. Finally, the writer commits the *kiss of death*, using *physician's assistant.*

This essay is for application to a graduate-level program at Baylor. The applicant has a master's degree, but the essay is long and drawn-out, full of grammatical errors, and very hard to follow. If I had to guess the education level of the writer, I would probably choose high school or below. Remember, communication is an essential quality we need to have as PAs, both verbal and written.

I sense the writer of this essay rushed to submit it on a deadline or treated it as just another box to check off in the application process.

The closing paragraph is also awkward. It should be a summation of why you want to become a PA. But, unfortunately, reading this essay, I don't think the writer ever answered the question, "*Why do you want to be a PA?*"

A word on the Passive Voice

I want to mention a way to improve your essays, make them easier to read and shorten sentences. You probably learned about the passive voice in high school but likely forgot about it. Yet, I see the passive voice used all of the time in the essays I review. If you want to make your essays clearer to read, learn to use the *active* voice in your writing.

What is passive voice?

Passive voice means that a *subject is a recipient of a verb's action.* Using the passive voice is not necessarily incorrect in certain situations, but for the most part, using the active voice will improve the readability of your essay.

Examples of passive voice:

Passive: *The book could not be read because…*
Active: *I could not read the book because…*

An active sentence has a different grammatical structure than a passive sentence. An active sentence begins with the *Subject* of the sentence; the *Subject* is the doer of the action. Below is the grammatical pattern:

Subject (the doer) + Verb (the action) + Object (the receiver of the action)

In the above active voice sentence example, the Subject is "I," the Verb is "read," and the Object is "the book." In the passive voice sentence example, the Object (The book) is first, the verb (read) is second, and there is no Subject.

Here are some more examples of passive voice sentences:

Passive: *My paper was reviewed by Kim.*
Active: *Kim reviewed my paper.*

Passive: *I was required to pass a difficult exam to obtain licensure as a professional counselor and complete 3,000 hours of supervised experience.*
Active: *I passed a difficult exam to obtain licensure as a professional counselor and complete 3,000 hours of supervised experience.*

Passive: *Since that time, I have been employed with Kingswood Pines Hospital for 3 years.*
Active: *I have worked at Kingwood Pines for the last 3 years.*

Passive: *Some friends and I were playing a little rough when Doris's toenail was accidentally ripped off.*
Active: *Doris's lost her toenail while some friends and I played a little rough.*

Notice in the above examples, the active voice sentence is always shorter than the passive voice sentence. This is because active voice limits the number of characters and makes the sentence more straightforward.

One way to identify passive verbs in your writing is to look for the "be" verbs. "Be" verbs include *be, am, are, is, been, was, and were.* Note that every example above contains a passive verb.

When reviewing your essay, look for sentences that include the passive voice. In addition, check every sentence for "be" verbs.

After attending an information session, I was struck by the program director's words that he views the program as a finishing school of sorts, where the students are fine polished until they can shine.